COUNTING MACROS FOR WEIGHT LOSS

THE BEGINNER'S GUIDE TO SUSTAINABLE WEIGHT LOSS BY BODY TYPE

ROBYN BROOKS

BROOKS BOOKS, LLC

PLEASE READ

INTRODUCTION

The distance between who I am and who I want to be is only separated by what I do! –Brian Solis

Weight loss: the two dreaded words that make most people shake in their boots. But what is it about the notion of losing weight that causes people to experience such bone-chilling and crippling anxiety? Could it be the fact that there seems to be such strict rules that accompany weight loss, or the fact that it seems like gaining weight is so easy but losing weight is so hard? Or is it the mere fact that the thought or need to lose weight often triggers discomfort, unhappiness, and feeling displeased with your own body? Whatever it is, losing weight or just being overall healthy is a pertinent part of life; it is important for staying physically, mentally, and emotionally sharp.

In the US alone, between 2017 and 2020, 41.9% of adults reportedly suffered from obesity (Centers for Disease Control and Prevention, 2021). This means that at some point, weight loss crossed the minds of almost 138 million people. What is most concerning, however, isn't how substantial this number is, but the fact that so many people are less than utterly and completely happy in their own bodies—the only body they will ever have.

It is time to change this!

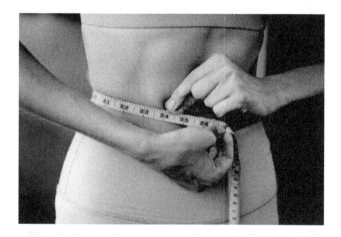

My name is Robyn Brooks, and much like you, I also once found myself unhappy with my body and my overall health. I began my weight loss journey a few years back, and I had to learn the process of effective weight loss the hard way. Between crash diets, binge eating, and nearly passing out from starving myself, I learned that none of those methods were effective in helping me lose weight, and instead of helping long term, they were doing my metabolism harm. With crash diets, I would eventually hit a wall, and in a short time, I would find myself back to the same weight, unhappy, and frustrated.

However, the more I delved into nutrition, the quicker I realized that summer bodies don't have to belong only in summer; these bodies are made in the kitchen. I was able to transform my body and my health simply by adhering to a macro-counting and meal-prepping lifestyle. And let me tell you, I wouldn't change it for the world! Not only did I find an effective weight loss solution that was designed for me and that catered to my body type, but I was finally able to achieve my weight loss goals. I felt better because I was getting all the nutrition I needed, and I had more energy to spend time with those most important to me—my family. Heck, I even became a Certified Nutritional Coach because I became excited about health and nutrition, and I wanted to share this excitement with as many people as possible.

The thing about being obese or even overweight is that it is no respecter of people. This means that adults from as young as 20 years old up to 60 years and older all suffer from obesity, and while it is less prevalent in younger people, it is still concerning, with 39.8% of young adults fighting obesity (Centers for Disease Control and Prevention, 2021). Additionally, it affects people from all cultural backgrounds, from all walks of life, and all socioeconomic statuses.

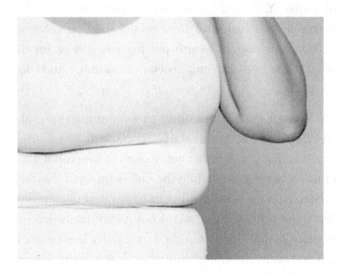

Being obese or overweight doesn't just stop you from living your life freely, but it also affects other areas of your life. People who are perceived as being overweight often feel discriminated against in the professional space, they are excluded from promotions and even from being hired, and this, in turn, affects their mental health (Yu, 2022). It has the power to propel them into depression and further into the hole from whence they are trying to escape.

Beyond the professional sphere, there are also the unique challenges that exist in families where people tend to have the same eating habits, whether those are healthy or unhealthy habits.

Obesity and being overweight is complex because there are a myriad of variables that you are constantly facing, whether it is from external people and factors or the onslaught that you internally subject yourself to on a daily basis. Internally, you may be plagued with concerns about health conditions that are associated with obesity or being overweight. You may be concerned about heart diseases, strokes and high blood pressure, diabetes, cancer, obstructive sleep apnea, and osteoarthritis. But it doesn't just end with physical ailments. You face concerns about how you look, how uncomfortable you feel, and how others may perceive you, all of which affect your mental health putting you at risk for developing depression, low self-esteem, social isolation, and low social adaptation.

Added to this are the external influences and the external variables that can affect the way you feel about yourself. There are emerging dietary trends that you can just never seem to keep up with, each new fad promising better results than the one before in a shorter time, but it all ultimately ends in you feeling unhappy and uncomfortable. The crash diets, the pills, and the weird not-meant-for-human-consumption alternatives that flood your feed on a daily basis leave you questioning if you really are doing enough to lose weight. But each leaves you feeling like it isn't going to work even before you start. This built-in bias tells you that you shouldn't even bother because quick-fix diets in the past never worked, so why would this one be any different?

Losing weight through extreme calorie deficit, or what I like to call "controlled starvation," is not beneficial because it takes away the nutritional value that our bodies so desperately yearn for. Losing muscle mass, not having energy, and being *hangry* all the time is great if you only care about a number on the scale, but when you realize that weight loss is far more than that number, the entire game changes.

And then, there is the variable of other people. I know body positivity begins with us, but blocking out the noise of people providing unsolicited and often useless weight loss advice, people telling you to just give up, and people promising you a miracle if you "just buy this supplement" can all make you feel overwhelmed. After all, weight loss isn't a journey that needs to be shared with the world unless *you* choose to do so.

I always say that the first person you need to please is yourself, and then you need to please your healthcare provider. You see, weight loss has this ripple effect where you feel good and look good on the outside, but your body also self-corrects on the inside. Things like blood sugar and blood pressure even out, cholesterol is lowered, and even though you don't see it, you will certainly feel the improvement.

But I know the pressing question is: How?

If you have been on a weight loss journey, or if you have struggled with your weight for a while, you may have come across something known as macro tracking. And while this may have been something you just brushed off as yet another ineffective fad, as something that is too confusing, or as something that costs an arm and a leg, it is actually an effective method of successfully achieving your weight loss goals... the science proves it!

In this book, I will guide you through a simple, yet detailed step-by-step system that teaches you the basics of macro tracking, how to identify your body's specific macro needs for effective weight loss, how to identify and understand your body type and how it intertwines with your dietary needs specifically for weight loss, and how to take all of this information and put it into use in a plan that allows you to lose weight while eating healthy and scrumptious meals.

And what can you, dear reader, expect in the future? Well, you may find yourself shedding pounds without restrictive diets; there will be no weight loss followed by weight gain once a "diet" ends because this isn't a diet—it's a lifestyle; meals that leave you happy and full and that help you lose and maintain weight are what you can expect.

So, let us go on this life-changing transformation together. It's going to be one heck of a ride!

1

INTRODUCING MACROS FOR WEIGHT LOSS

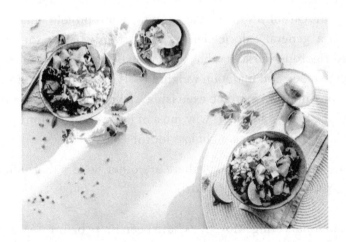

Whether or not you have heard of macros, a good place for us to start is defining the terminology. This lays the foundation and helps you understand the "what" before implementing the "how."

In this chapter, we are going to look at what exactly macros are, why counting macros are beneficial for weight loss and weight maintenance, and we will take a little deep dive into why so many diets fail.

Also, an important aspect of weight loss is goal setting. I can't tell you how many times I have searched the words: "How to lose weight" and actually found people making promises that their techniques would work. . . in 10 days. If I knew then what I know now, I would have been fully aware that all I was doing was setting myself up for disappointment because these were entirely and completely unrealistic goals.

You may find yourself wondering why you aren't losing any weight. I can't tell you how many times I have stood on the scale, feeling slightly confident, only to see the number staring back at me and feeling utterly and entirely devastated. "How is this even possible?" I would ask myself with tears in my eyes. There are a couple of reasons why this occurs. I am sure on your weight loss journey, you have seen the emphasis that is placed on dietary restrictions such as cutting down your carbohydrate intake, upping your protein intake, and being in a general calorie deficit. This, coupled with the recommended rigorous workouts that you are expected to do, can make it difficult to reach and maintain weight loss. A focus on trying to eat as little as possible and extreme exercising isn't enough to help you lose weight long term, and that is why most of these changes don't permanently help you on your weight loss journey.

What we fail to realize is that there are other factors that influence weight loss. These are (Jomol, 2021):

1. Emotional eating: Most of us have been there before — we overeat because we are upset, or we devour too many chocolates because we are extremely stressed. Ignoring the role that our emotions play in our eating habits is like ignoring our oven when it comes to cooking. They play an essential role, and it isn't only bad emotions that affect our eating habits. Even happiness and celebrations can lead us to overindulge.
2. Being impatient: No one wants to lose weight over six months. We all want to lose weight immediately. But this

goes hand-in-hand with setting unrealistic goals for ourselves. If you want to lose 10 pounds in a month, the chances of you giving up when you see that you've only lost five pounds is huge. However, if you had set a goal to lose five pounds, you will feel accomplished when you do lose those five pounds, and you will be motivated to continue on your weight loss journey.

3. False body image view: Your body might never look like the people on the front cover of a magazine. When you change your body image, you realize that each person has a different body structure. Some people have wide hips, others have broad shoulders, and each type is beautiful. But it does mean that your attempts to look like a front cover model are going to be futile, especially if your body types aren't the same.

4. Stress: Much like our emotions, stress also plays a big role in our weight gain and weight loss. Stress causes a rise in a hormone called cortisol, and studies have shown that regularly elevated cortisol levels lead to an increased appetite and weight gain. You could spend hours in the gym and eat hardly anything at all, but depending on how much stress your body is under and how your body copes with stress, you may not see any results at all.

5. Sedentary lifestyle: If you work out for 20 minutes in a day and spend the other 23 hours and 40 minutes on the sofa eating junk food, the chances of you losing weight are zero to none. This is an extreme and unrealistic example, but it is important to make sure you reduce a sedentary lifestyle (if you lead one) to see the most results in your weight loss.

6. Diet pills: What if I told you that most diet pills don't help you with weight loss but rather just reduce your water weight, rendering them ineffective for actual fat loss? This sometimes means that people depend on diet pills to lose weight when diet pills aren't effective for actual long term weight loss.

7. Gut health: Our gut plays an important part in our overall health. If we don't take care of our gut health, we will quickly find that we have reached a plateau in weight loss no matter how little food we eat.

With this in mind, let's take a look at macros and how they can play an important role in your weight loss journey.

What Are Macros?

For the longest time, I would shy away from anything that had to do with counting, whether it was counting calories, counting and measuring your meals, or everything else that went along with a number attached to it. I always thought it would take away from the enjoyment of eating. That was until I learned about macronutrients.

Macronutrients, or macros as you will often see referred to in this book, are the nutrients that our bodies need in large doses. Now, even if you haven't heard of macronutrients before, I am almost entirely certain that you have heard of carbohydrates, proteins, and fats. Guess what? These three comprise macronutrients.

Each of these macros is measured in grams, and they differ slightly from each other in terms of how many calories they each have per gram. This will, in turn, affect the nutrient density of the macro. For example, fats are considered more nutrient dense than protein and carbs because, for each gram, they have more than double the number of calories than proteins and carbs. Fat has about nine calories for every gram, but carbs and proteins have about four calories for every gram (Horton, 2023).

The way we can look at the notion of macronutrients is that each day, we have an allotted calorie budget. For example, in a day, depending on your weight loss goals, your body type, and the type of workouts and exercises you are doing, you will have a certain amount of calories you would need to consume (for weight loss, your calorie intake would need to be less than your bodies calorie or energy expenditure at rest because breathing, a beating heart, and a working brain all uses calories). Depending on how many calories you need to be taking in, a percentage needs to be dedicated to fats, proteins, and carbs, as well as to micronutrients, which opposed to macronutrients, are what your body needs in smaller doses such as fiber, calcium, and other vitamins and minerals.

To further break this down, you should consume, and your diet should be comprised of between 10% to 35% of protein, 45% to 65% of carbs, and 20% to 35% of good fats (Horton, 2023).

Of the many factors that need to be considered and that will influence your calorie intake, it will not only include your weight loss goals and how active you are in a day, but it will also include your age, gender, height, weight, and your basal metabolic rate (BMR).

In many cases, people find it more effective to count macros than counting calories alone. This is because you don't need to assign a single number to everything you eat, which inevitably makes eating a chore rather than something enjoyable. Once you figure out the percentage of macros you should be targeting, it all gets easier from there because all you have to do is stay within your target. This means that you can eat anything and everything, so long as it stays within the limits you have established for yourself. Granted, it isn't about quality over quantity, and it literally boils down to how much of each macro you eat rather than what type of macro you are eating. However, if you have a goal of feeling better and improving your health, quality matters.

Food Sources for Macros

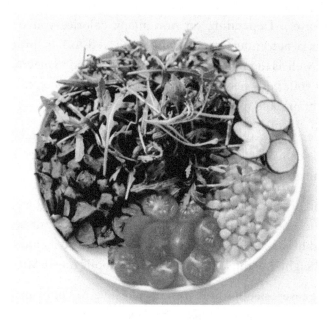

So where can you get your macros from? Whether or not you can eat whatever you want, it is up to you to decide how you are going to get your intake of macros. I always recommend going for quality over quantity. There is a common saying that states you should have 80% healthy foods and 20% indulgences, and when counting macros, the same can be said.

There are many sources that you can get high quality macros from. You can get carbs from:

- whole grains
- lentils
- a variety of fruit and vegetables

Proteins can come from:

- fish
- chicken
- red meat
- beans
- lentils
- egg whites

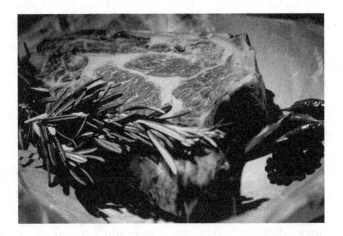

Fats are the tricky ones because they are nutrient-rich, which means that a little goes a long way. Also, there are trans fats, saturated fats, and unsaturated fats. Trans fats have no health benefits and should be avoided at all costs, and saturated fats can lead to higher risks of heart disease and high cholesterol and should therefore be limited (Nelson, 2021). You can get healthy fats from:

- nuts and nut butters
- dairy products
- vegetable oils
- fish
- seeds

Macros not only give you a way to limit your food intake, but it also gives you the freedom to enjoy what you are eating and allows you to eat almost anything, provided you stay within your macro limits.

Why Most Diets Fail

I know, sometimes you may wonder if you are the one doing something wrong because no matter what you do, no diet seems to work. Do you want to know why you feel this way? The short answer is that diets are temporary, but lifestyle changes are permanent. Diets tell you to restrict your intake and limit what you eat, but lifestyle changes tell you that you can have everything in moderation.

But let's look at this in a different light. Our bodies have natural stress responses to external stimuli. Our stress responses are usually hormonal responses that alert our bodies of danger. In a primal form, it evokes a fight or flight mechanism. Our body does whatever it needs to do to survive. However, we aren't in a primal phase of life, so our stress response pushes us to work through deadlines and other similar aspects to do whatever it takes to stay alive. Researchers found that in mice, dieting makes the brain more sensitive to stress, meaning that it inclines one's susceptibility to stress and it makes you crave the rewards of high-fat and high-calorie foods (Arnold, 2010). Dieting basically evokes the same response as what prompts us to eat an entire tub of ice cream after a breakup or a difficult day at work. Dieting places our bodies under stress and makes us seek junk food to soothe that stress.

Aside from this internal response to dieting, there are other reasons why diets may fail. The first reason may be a strange one to consider, and that is using willpower instead of science to control hunger. Have you ever heard someone tell you to embrace your hunger when you are dieting? Well, willpower (which is used to stop yourself from eating) can inadvertently be seen by your body as starvation. This happens because your body doesn't know that you are trying to lose weight, and if you are not getting the correct levels of nutrients it puts the body into survival mode. Therefore, our body kicks into effect mechanisms to obviously keep us from starving to death, and it increases our hunger and cravings and also slows down our metabolism, so we don't burn through energy as fast. Using the science-based approach of counting macros ensures your body will get the nutrients it needs in the proper balance. This alone keeps the body from thinking you are starving.

The next reason is that not all calories are created the same. This is also one of the reasons I view counting macros as better than counting calories. Macros come from specific sources, but calories come from everything. It's hard to eat "bad" proteins since, in most cases, bad proteins don't exist. However, not all calories are created equally. There are some that spike your insulin and cause your body to store fat, and there are others that sustain your body and promote weight loss. Focusing on trying to take in a specific number of calories but not paying any mind to the source of those calories is a recipe for disaster.

Another seemingly shocking reason why diets may fail is that some people think they need to cut out fats. This is not true, especially when you consider that there are a wide variety of healthy fats that exist out there. Eating more fats than carbs has the possibility to increase your metabolism by up to 300 calories per day (Hyman, 2014). It is also a false notion that fat will cause you to gain weight, and the truth is, it is usually sugar that causes your weight to go up. Now, when I say that fat is good for weight loss, I don't mean that you should eat the greasiest and fattest burger that exists. Instead, you need to choose healthy fats such as avocado, nuts, eggs, meat, and omega-3 fatty acids.

The next reason that diets may not work is because of unseen health and medical reasons. If we consider that our bodily functions are controlled by unseen variables, a lot of internal workings may cause a diet to be ineffective. There are some people who exercise everyday, and they do extremely intense workouts, and by all accounts, they eat extremely healthy meals, but for some reason, they are stuck and unable to get beyond a certain point in their weight loss journey. This isn't because they are doing something wrong, but rather that their internal functions are not working at an optimal level. These could be things such as diabetes or insulin resistance, inflammation or poor gut health, food allergies, a build-up of toxins, and even thyroid problems.

In many of these cases, many people don't go to the doctor to test their health because they may otherwise feel fine, but in fact, they are facing blocks in their weight loss journey that can only be treated by a medical professional.

Finally, another glaringly obvious reason why diets may not work is that they don't have a long-term plan in place. How many times have you decided that you are going to start a diet on Monday, but when Monday rolls around, the pantry is packed with snacks and nothing that will be beneficial to your diet? This is the position I found myself in many times. I also told myself that I couldn't start a diet with a cupboard full of junk food, and so I convinced myself that I needed to eat all the junk food before I started a diet. To say that I didn't have a plan would be a staggering understatement.

The previous factors all fall into two major categories: our physiology (which includes our metabolism, calorie intake, our hormones, the way our body responds to certain foods, and the type of macros we consume) and our psychology (which includes things like our willpower, mindset, motivation, the way we perceive food, our relationship with food, and our overall mood).

Establishing the Ideal Weight Loss Goals

The best way for a "diet" to be successful is, in fact, if you don't follow a diet at all. I know this may sound insane, but there are two things that you need to consider: weight loss isn't just about dropping the number on the scale but is rather about being healthy (weight loss will follow suit), and weight loss also comes with a lifestyle change. Weight loss isn't a "just for now until I reach my goal weight" situation, and it most certainly isn't a quick fix. Instead, it is about making long-lasting behavioral changes.

One of the best ways to achieve this healthy lifestyle and to make long-lasting behavioral changes is to establish the ideal weight loss goals. Goals not only give you purpose and something to work toward, but they also make you accountable, whether it is to someone else or to yourself.

So how do you set effective weight loss goals, and I mean specific to weight loss? Well, you first need to know where you are starting. Many people want to fit into a size four, but they currently wear a size twelve. Would this mean that they need to lose weight or that they may have unrealistic expectations of their body type and goals? I once read something that made me laugh because of how true it was. It said, "I miss the time I thought I was fat, but I wasn't actually fat because now I am actually fat, and I would do anything to go back to the fake fat version of myself."

Before you set goals (realistic goals, that is), you first need to know where you are starting and where you are hoping to go from here. While each person is different, there are a variety of factors that would influence whether or not you should be pursuing weight loss. A good rule of thumb for anyone trying to figure out if they need to lose weight and set weight loss goals for themselves are if they have a Body Mass Index (BMI) greater than 25, if their waist circumference is greater than 35 inches for women and 40 in. for men, and if their waist to hip ratio is greater than 0.8 for women and 1.0 for men (Waehner, 2022).

If there are people who want to do more about their health, but they don't necessarily fit into a criteria to lose weight, there are always other goals that they can set for themselves, such as increasing their muscle tone, flexibility, and overall health. But for the purpose of this book, we are focusing solely on weight loss.

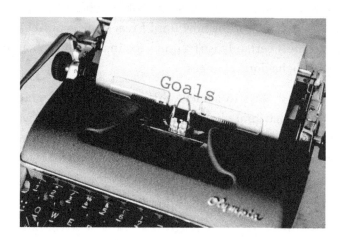

So how do you set goals for weight loss? Well, let me share with you a blueprint for setting goals, not just for weight loss, but for every other facet of your life. These are known as SMART goals and are defined as follows (Waehner, 2022):

- **Specific:** This means giving yourself exact weight amounts or inches that you are hoping to lose.
- **Measurable:** If you don't have a starting point from which to work, how will you keep track of your progress? Whether this is a starting weight, a starting measurement, or before pictures, always be sure to document your starting point so your goal can be measured and further broken down if need be.
- **Attainable:** Your goals need to be something that you have the tools, resources, and physical ability to achieve. You can't set a goal that requires you to lose more weight than is healthy or possible for your body. Setting shorter goals that add up to one big goal over time is a great way to ensure your goals are attainable.

- **Realistic:** While in life you are usually encouraged to be ambitious; this is not encouraged during weight loss. Over-ambitious weight loss goals are a recipe for disaster because your chances of achieving them are minimized. One to two pounds per week is considered a realistic goal for weight loss.
- **Time-bound:** A goal isn't a goal without a deadline. Personally, my motivation is much higher when I know I have a deadline than when I leave things to chance. Establishing a timeline, even if it isn't precise, allows you to push yourself through difficult days and adapt according to what is realistic and what you can achieve in a given time.

With these concepts in mind, it is important that you are fully prepared and equipped to lose weight. You need to be ready for the hard work because this will make sure that you don't give up before you even start seeing results, and it also allows you to establish consistency. Remember, motivation will come and go—being healthy means working toward your goals whether or not you are in the mood or have the motivation.

Setting realistic goals and being reasonable about your time frame are key components to a healthy weight loss regimen. While rapid weight loss may sound great and will probably wow all those around you when you shed the weight slowly, you are more likely to maintain the weight loss.

Summary

- Macros are the macronutrients your body needs in large doses and are made up of fats, proteins, and carbohydrates.
- Most diets fail because they are short-term and have the potential for placing our bodies under high stress. Our physiology and psychology also impact our ability to effectively lose weight and need to be considered when we plan our weight loss plans.

- Creating SMART goals is a great way to achieve our weight loss goals.

Now that we have a foundational understanding of why some diets work and why others don't, we can now delve into a detailed and scientific understanding of counting macros. It's not just another miracle diet but an effective weight loss tool.

2

THE SCIENCE BEHIND MACROS

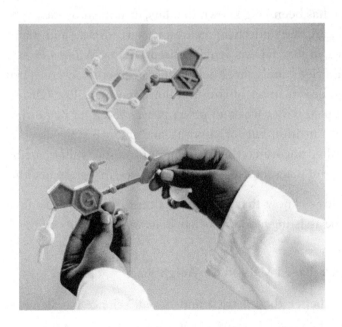

I am sure that, just like me, you have heard of "miracle diets." You know the type I'm talking about. The ones that make unrealistic promises or the ones that you know for a fact are way too good to be true. Counting macros defies the notion of a miracle diet in almost every way. While these miracle diets offer you fast fat-burning results, they often lead to you feeling hungry and frustrated. On the other hand, counting macros means you're playing the long game. It's not going to be quick, but you will see results, you will be healthier, and you will enjoy one of the best parts of life—food.

Keeping track of and counting your intake of macronutrients isn't a miracle diet but is instead deeply rooted in scientific fact. The reality is that our bodies are designed to take in certain amounts of carbs, proteins, and fats for them to maintain their nutritional balance. It works in a scientific balance that, if counted correctly and in the right way, can aid in weight loss and maintain weight management. Remember, we are not working on short-term goals but on long-term health.

While it has been long known that fats, or unhealthy fats, to be more specific, are the underlying cause of heart disease and many other ailments, in 1827, fat was actually discovered by William Prout to be a macronutrient, and since then, it has been studied and purified to find the best manner of consumption for weight loss (Olson, 1998). Fat, coupled with carbs and proteins, was found to be pertinent not only for nutrition but for survival, and upon further assessment, it was further uncovered that there are nutritional values attributed to each type of macronutrient and that fats can, in fact, be healthy.

Little did we know, that more than a century later, these discoveries would be assisting modern society in its weight loss journey.

A Science-Based Method for Weight Loss

What is better than a tried and tested, science-based method for weight loss? The last thing anyone wants is empty promises, so if I have science-backed facts, you can surely bet that I am going to look deeper into it. And that is exactly what I did with counting macros. In a basic understanding, the reason why people count macros is so they can understand where their calorie intake is coming from. When you're counting macros, your perspective is different than when compared to counting calories. When you count calories, you are given a number that is the daily intake you can consume, and in so doing, people tend to fill that number of allotted calories with anything and everything, whether or not it is healthy or nutrient-rich foods. In this way, you may find people who are overweight but also severely malnourished. This may not make sense, but when you consider that their calorie intake was filled with food that posed little nutritional benefit to them, you can see how they gained weight and were so unhealthy.

However, when you are counting macros, you look at the entire process in a different way and from a different perspective. Yes, in the same way, you have a certain number of allotted calories in a day that you can consume, but instead of just filling it with anything and everything, you are being conscious and aware of what you are consuming. When you look at it in this way, your allotted calorie intake isn't filled with just anything but is very purposeful to make sure your body is getting exactly what it needs. Counting macros, therefore, helps you keep track of what you are eating, where it is coming from, and how the food interacts with and impacts your body.

But this still begs the question of how counting macros can help you lose weight. Well, this simple answer is that counting macros allows you to maintain nutritional value in the food that you eat rather than "spending" your calories on food that has little nutritional value. This is how you find people who are "skinny fat" or who may not look like it, but they suffer from diabetes and high cholesterol.

At first, when you put this into practice, it may seem like a lot of work. This is especially true when you consider that counting the macros doesn't tell you what you are supposed to eat. Consider a breakfast that consists of 15g of protein, 25g of carbs, and 5g of fat. This may seem like a great and balanced meal in terms of macronutrients, but this meal could be protein powder mixed with flour and a scoop of butter. That doesn't even sound appetizing, let alone healthy.

Instead of creating strange combinations, when you count macros, you are going to consider the foods you already eat. By focusing on the macronutrients that are present in your meals, you have better control over what you eat as opposed to making meals based on macronutrients. On the other hand, you may find it easier to meal plan and prep based on macronutrients. You must find what works best for you. There is a simple and straightforward way of assessing what macros are present in your meal. The nutritional information on any packaged product gives you information about what macros are in the food. Once you familiarize yourself with looking at what is in your food, counting macros becomes much easier.

Counting macros also helps you assess exactly what you are putting in your body. If you are eating two meals, and both have 28g of protein, one may be healthier than the other because one may have more sugar than the other. Counting macros will enable you to recognize healthier food choices, which will in turn improve your overall health.

Now, what happens when nutritional information isn't available? You don't really see nutritional information tables on fresh produce or on many other whole foods for that matter. Luckily, every food item has a nutritional value that scientists have studied in detail to determine the amount of macro and micronutrients in the item (Fry, 2018). You can easily find trackers and mobile applications that will tell you exactly what nutrients are in most food items.

Counting Macros: Does It Work?

There are two ways of answering this: the short way and the long way. The short answer, quite simply stated, is yes, counting macronutrients do work not just for weight loss but for overall weight management too. Now, let's look at the long answer, where we delve into how it works.

At its foundation, counting macros work in the same way as counting calories because it works based on energy input and energy expenditure. We have already seen that everything in our body requires energy. Even our hearts beating and breathing air in and out use energy. But what makes macro tracking much easier is that you get to lose weight in a healthy way.

You see, losing weight is greatly assisted by your muscle mass. When you lose weight, it is almost a guarantee that you may lose muscle mass with your fat. But one way to stop this, or at least minimize the loss of muscle mass, is to count macros. When you are actively and correctly counting macros, you can better develop your calorie or energy "spend," whether you choose to do so on a daily or weekly basis. If you want to lose weight, you can be in an energy deficit while still consuming the exact macronutrients that you need. If you need to gain weight, you can do so in a healthy way, and if you want to maintain weight, you can also monitor and regulate your macro intake.

Counting macros also makes it easy for you to keep track of where your macros may be lacking on a specific day. If you are a bit low on your protein intake, you can have some steak, chicken, or low-fat cottage cheese, and if you are low on fat, you can have an avocado or some nuts. This makes it easier to get nutrient-dense food rather than just filling your calories with foods that aren't beneficial to your body (Hunt, 2021).

Finding the Balance in Your Diet

We are all about balanced diets and losing weight at a healthy pace. I can say that with confidence because I know you wouldn't be here reading this book if health wasn't your priority. We have already established that counting macros makes it easier for you to maintain your health and nutritional balance as opposed to counting calories, because macros help you maintain quality in the number of calories you are eating. In a nutshell, counting macros allows you to control your calories in a nutritionally healthy way.

It is so important to find health and balance because if it were all about weight loss, it would be easy to jump on the next diet fad, drop those pounds almost instantly, but suffer from inexplicable symptoms because you didn't pursue better health with the weight loss.

As I began studying to become a nutritional coach and I got a better understanding of how nutrition worked, I was better able to understand the circumstances of two very different friends who both found themselves suffering from symptoms of malnourishment. The first was a woman who was 34 years old and who always seemed to be fixated on her weight. Her weight generally fluctuated, and when it was high, she would do whatever it took to get her weight back down. This often included her eating as little as possible and taking in as few calories as possible in the hopes of dropping some pounds. There were some days when she would hardly eat anything at all. The strangest thing was that her kids were always well-fed, she had the financial means and time to cook nutritious meals, and she would have never realized that she had a nutrient deficiency if she hadn't started experiencing symptoms that prompted her to see a doctor.

She began experiencing severe hair loss, far more than usual, and would shed so much hair that bald spots were beginning to appear on her head, she had a cut on her leg that refused to heal, but the last straw that prompted her to see a doctor was when she stubbed her toe on the coffee table and ended up fracturing two bones in her foot.

You see, malnutrition presents with symptoms that people often fail to realize are not normal. Things such as hair loss, tooth decay, depression and anxiety, burning sensations in your extremities, wounds that take a long to heal, bone pain and a loss of bone density, irregular heartbeats, poor vision, and the onset of illnesses such as high blood pressure, cholesterol, diabetes, cancers, and strokes can all be caused by malnutrition.

On the flip side of this coin, I also had a friend who was obese. He was 27 years old, worked from home, lived by himself, and he lived off fast food, junk food, and soda. However, he presented with many of the same symptoms as the acquaintance I mentioned earlier. He was balding at this young age, he had severe joint pain, he suffered from chronic, extreme fatigue despite sleeping for more than 10 hours a day, and he could never seem to focus on the task at hand. Despite being obese, he was malnourished because everything that he put in his body had minimal nutritional value.

In both cases, with major adjustments to their diets, both were able to maintain a healthy weight and lose weight respectively in a healthy way. There is a false notion that accompanies the word "malnutrition" in that we think it exists only in some parts of the world. Malnutrition can plague anyone who doesn't give their body what it so desperately yearns for. Counting macros is one surefire way of making sure you get in the nutrients you need.

So how can you find the nutrients you need on a daily basis? Well, we are going to investigate what *good* sources of *healthy* carbs, fats, and proteins are.

Carbohydrates

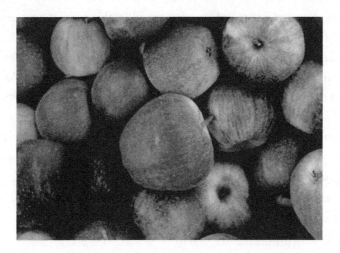

In many diets, carbs are almost seen as a bad word that should be avoided, like the plague. But the reality is that carbs form an important part of a balanced diet. Now, the reason carbs have developed such a bad reputation is because of an overgeneralization that has come about. Allow me to break the details down for you: There are two types of carbs, namely simple carbohydrates and complex carbohydrates. Pretty much as the name suggests, simple carbs are the ones we usually find readily available in natural foods, such as the sugar in honey and dairy products. Because simple carbs are *simple*, it means that they are quite easy for the body to break down; they can be used as a quick source of energy.

Complex carbs are the carbs that have a more complex molecular structure meaning that they aren't as quickly broken down by the body. These are foods such as fiber and whole grains, and they are usually the foods that keep you fuller for longer. Because they have a slower release of energy, they stay in your body longer and provide you with energy over a long period. This is why wholesome meals with a lot of vegetables keep your hunger satisfied for so long. Fiber, beans, many root vegetables, and grains are all great sources of complex carbs.

Now, here is where things get a bit misinterpreted. There are simple and complex carbs that, when consumed in the correct amounts, are extremely beneficial to your body, your nutrition, your health, and even your weight loss journey. These are the carbs that are referred to as unrefined; you eat them as you find them; they are whole foods that have not been processed or adjusted much (if at all) from their natural state. On the flip side, you have refined carbs. These are the food items that have been so severely processed that they are stripped of almost all nutritional value, and they are the leading cause of obesity, weight gain, and diabetes. This is because despite being void of any real nutritional value, they carry the same number of calories. Fast food, processed chips, and candy are all major contributors to refined carbs (Bhupathiraju & Hu, n.d.).

Fats

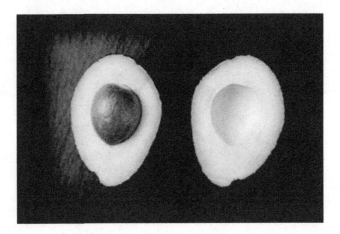

The next macronutrient that, just by name, can send shivers down the spine of anyone hoping to lose a couple of pounds is *fats*. Don't let a little fat in your diet scare you. If you are focused on improving your health, the truth is, you need fats. Fats are necessary for your body to absorb vitamins A, D, E, and K. Just in the same way that there are healthy and unhealthy carbs, there are also healthy and unhealthy fats. Stick with the healthy fats that fit into your macronutrient goals. Unsaturated fats are the fats that are healthy and good for your body, of which Omega-3 is one. On the other end of the spectrum are trans fats which are unhealthy fats, the ones that are extremely processed. But there are healthy fats that can be found in (Vetter, 2022):

- fish, which are oily and are rich in Omega-3 fatty acids
- avocados
- full-fat dairy products (in moderation)
- seeds
- nuts

Proteins

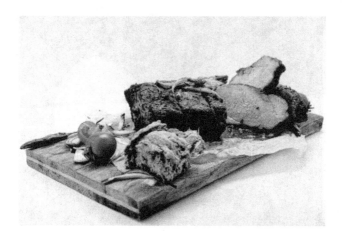

Proteins are a superfood that all humans need to survive. They not only promote weight loss because of the unique role they play in muscle development and maintenance, but they also feed the muscles that you don't always consider as muscles, such as your heart and brain. Protein also works to repair cell damage which is essentially what happens when you go to the gym and work out. That is why protein is so important and works hand in hand with fitness.

There are two sources of protein, namely plant protein and animal protein. In most cases, animal proteins are complete proteins that have all nine essential amino acids present, and incomplete proteins may be missing one or more essential amino acids. Essential amino acids are the amino acids your body doesn't produce, so you must get them from foods. Plants are incomplete proteins, so if you're on a plant-based diet, you will need to eat a variety of plant proteins in order to get certain amino acids that are absent in one food from another food source.

Both animal and plant proteins are great for your body, for cell repair, and for forming an extremely important part of your diet and nutrition. You can find protein in:

- meat
- chicken
- fish
- tofu
- legumes
- beans
- nuts
- eggs

How Macros Affect Weight Loss

Our bodies are all about balance. When you consider counting calories and macros, it's all about balancing the scale and putting out exactly what you have taken in, depending on your goals. The same goes for the ratio of macros you consume, depending on what your goals are.

Just because you aren't counting calories doesn't mean you're allowed free reign on the amount of protein, carbs, and fat that you eat. Instead, when you are focusing on macronutrients, you will find that you may get fuller a lot faster because of the wholesome foods you are eating, and without even realizing it, your calorie intake may be drastically reduced (Van De Walle, 2018).

There have been studies that sought to assess what was the optimal macronutrient ratio for weight loss, but essentially, the research found that weight loss is extremely achievable if you keep your ratios in the 10%-35% proteins, 45%-65% carbs, and 20%-35% fats range. This was especially true when measured long term (Gardner et al., 2018; Sacks et al., 2009). Ideally, you will want to take in a ratio that you can stick with and adjust the ratio to your personal body type because consistency matters. But remember this still means you should be taking in healthy carbs, fats, and proteins, and ultimately, you are striving for a calorie deficit to lose weight.

There is also the notion of "If It Fits Your Macros," or IIFYM, which is an idea that asks what you can eat while still seeing results (obviously depending on what your goals are). This serves the notion that you are allowed to eat anything and everything so long as your calorie intake is controlled and you get a well-distributed percentage of macronutrients in that meal, whether it is an indulgence or a healthy meal.

When it comes to counting macros, it is safe to say that it is all about quality over quantity. If you compare a brownie to a salad rich in vegetables, in terms of IIFYM, both are fine for you to consume, but in the greater scheme of things, the brownie doesn't carry much quality. Instead, one has a higher calorie value, and the other has a lower calorie value, but the vegetable rich salad is the one that really provides you with the macronutrients that are needed. In terms of counting macros, the salad would be a better choice for your body because the way your body would process and respond to each would be different.

Protein for Weight Loss

We have already discussed how wonderful protein is for weight loss and muscle maintenance, but it is also beneficial, particularly for weight loss, in other ways. First, protein affects our body at a hormonal level. Not only does it regulate hormones, but it also reduces the hormones that trigger the feeling of hunger. Next, when you consider that our bodies burn calories during normal functions, such as our hearts beating and metabolizing food, once again, protein serves as a beneficial macronutrient because the body burns more calories when digesting protein. Protein also boosts your metabolism and keeps you fuller longer by reducing your appetite, causing you to consume fewer calories, and it reduces your cravings for snacks.

In a nutshell, while there is no hard and fast ratio for optimal macronutrient consumption that will encourage weight loss, taking in enough protein is a surefire way to make sure you indirectly consume fewer calories and that you lose weight in a healthy way.

Summary

- Counting macronutrients is not just a fad but is based on science, which allows you to lose weight but to do so in a healthy way.
- There are whole food sources of each macronutrient that allow your body to consume these nutrients in a healthy way that is optimized and easy for your body to break down and process.
- There is no particular ratio that proves best for weight loss, but you can never go wrong with consuming enough protein!

In the next chapter, we are going to delve into body types, and how they can affect our weight loss attempts.

3

UNDERSTANDING YOUR BODY TYPE
AND HOW IT AFFECTS WEIGHT LOSS

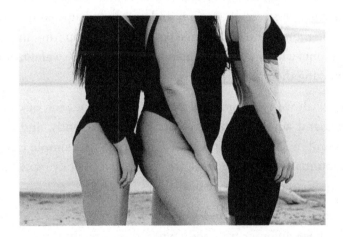

One of the unique beauties of this world is that we are all different. While this is absolutely true in terms of personality, preferences, and physical appearance, it is also true for body types. From the expected differences that we have in terms of hormonal changes, to where we are and what we are doing, to our mindset and our mental standpoint at any given point, in a world with more than seven billion people; there are rarely more than a handful of people at any given time who are dealing with the exact same circumstances.

Let us look at a hypothetical situation. If we were to take 100 people of varying ethnicities, genders, societal outlooks, and eating habits, and if we put these individuals into a room and each of these people ate the exact same thing in terms of food type and quantity; if we did this over an extended period, each person would look entirely different. At our very foundation, we all have different metabolic rates that are affected by several internal and environmental factors.

This is, in fact, something that came up in a group of my friends when we were discussing how we struggled with weight after having children. Some of us had gained weight and struggled to lose it, and others seemed to stay thin no matter what they ate. The change in routine and caring for little ones came with new stresses and new circumstances to deal with. This, coupled with the fact that we had different work challenges to deal with, meant that some of us began processing our stress by eating, and we ended up gaining weight. Sadly, the moms who had gained weight were comparing themselves to the moms who quickly returned to their pre-baby weight, and they were making themselves feel miserable.

What I wish we could have all understood is that each of us handle changes and adjust to the stressors of life differently, and that our bodies and metabolisms are entirely different. The simple fact is that at the foundation of our beings, we have different body types, and our body types affect the way we burn and store fat.

It's important for you to understand what we didn't understand, that despite these differences in body types, there are ways to work toward your weight loss goals that play into the advantages of your particular body type, no matter what it is.

There may be instances where you feel like no matter how much you diet, you can't seem to lose weight. But the reality is that once you learn what body type you are, the weight loss and health game changes.

What Is a Body Type?

I know that there are many people who shy away from visiting dieticians, nutritionists, weight loss coaches, and even personal trainers, and they are under the impression that there is no way that weight loss can be personalized to them and their circumstances. However, in actual fact, in the 1940s, a medical doctor by the name of William H. Sheldon devised the notion of somatotypes, or what we have come to know as different body types (Center for Wellness Without Borders, n.d.). We will delve into each of the body types that exist, but basically, there are three different body types that people fall into. Nutritionists, dieticians, fitness trainers, and doctors are able to personalize health and weight loss programs for individuals because they have studied and learned the science behind each body type and how each body type metabolizes and burns energy.

For the most part, people generally fall into one of three somatotypes, namely ectomorph, endomorph, or mesomorph. People may not fit neatly into each body type, but it is a general derivative of our genetics. Your body type is more of a generalization, but it is the body composition that we are all expected to have. While our body types are pretty much set in stone and cannot be altered, there are also physiological and psychological determining factors that contribute to one's body type.

It is also important to realize that body types exist on a spectrum. This means that even those who belong to a similar body type may not have the exact same metabolism and may not be able to process food or weight loss in the exact same way. Dr. Sheldon also theorized that because body types were predetermined genetically, in most cases, they will also affect and contribute to one's personality.

As body types were studied further, in recent times, the spectrum analogy of body types has gained greater traction and only differs from Dr. Sheldon's understanding in one way: Instead of our body type influencing our personality and our physiological and psychological composition, modern science rather believes that our current body type can fluctuate (existing on a spectrum), and that can, in turn, affect our physiology and psychology (Payne, 2020).

Let us delve deeper into these three different body types and how you can identify which body type you are.

Ectomorph

If we consider the previous story, the mom who seemed to stay small and tiny no matter what she ate, she would be an example of an ectomorph body type. While this friend may have been very tiny, there is often a misconception that size is an indicator of health. She would eat fast foods and junk foods, but she continued to have a lower muscle mass, and in fact, it is extremely hard for ectomorphs to gain muscle. This is not a flaw in the system but is rather the natural composition of an ectomorph body type.

These individuals have a very lean and delicate body type because their shoulders and hips are much narrower in relation to their height, but their limbs appear much longer. They also have small muscles when compared to the length of their bones, and they tend to have fast metabolisms. This makes it difficult for them to not only gain weight but to gain muscle as well. In many cases, people with this body type may end up being something known as "skinny fat" because they can eat everything, no matter how unhealthy it may be, and they do not gain weight. While they look slim on the outside, the harm is done internally when their cholesterol goes up, their blood sugar rises, and they face high blood pressure.

Endomorph

Seemingly, the counterpart of the ectomorph body type exists the endomorph body type. Once again, looking at the same scenario, many body types represent the endomorph body type because people seem to gain weight far too easily. However, easily gaining weight is not the only characteristic of the endomorph body type. People who have this body type tend to be seen as the soft and round body type. This isn't because they are just walking marshmallows, but rather because they don't appear to have a great muscle mass, and they appear to have their fat concentrated around their waist areas. This, coupled with the fact that their limbs appear to be relatively short when compared to the rest of their body, gives a greater appearance of a rounded body figure.

In most cases, people who have this body type generally seem to have a slower metabolism, and they appear to gain weight faster and lose it slower. They usually end up extremely frustrated about their weight because it often feels like one day of not sticking to their extremely strict diet leads to them gaining weight.

Mesomorph

Finally, there's the mesomorph body type. The mesomorph body type is the one that seems to be given to the favorites in the world. I am absolutely kidding, of course, but these are the people who seem to need to put in no effort to get a wonderful physique. Mesomorphs have a generally medium structure, and they appear to have an inverted triangular body shape, with their shoulders being slightly broader than the hips. They also have a generally athletic build and both weight gain or weight loss happen quite easily, whether it is muscle or fat (gain or loss).

These are the individuals who are not only naturally inclined to be athletic and play sports, but they are also generally good at sports as well.

Through these descriptions, it is usually quite easy for people to determine what their body type is. However, if you do decide to head to a doctor or a nutritionist, they may do further tests on your hormone levels and on your metabolism that may allow them to more accurately determine what body type you may have.

Despite the body type you fit in, you can still actively work toward improving your health. Through exercise and a healthy diet, you will find your body moving along the spectrum of whichever body type you fit in. Remember that at the foundation of health is consistency. Those with an endomorph body type, who appear to be rounded in the center, can minimize their weight gain by exercising regularly and making sure they consume a healthier diet. This means that you aren't sentenced to one body type for life. If you put in the work, you could definitely see results in moving along the spectrum that exists within body types.

How Body Types Affect Weight Loss

Now that we know a bit about each body type, the pressing question is: How does it affect weight loss? As has been the theme throughout this book thus far, in terms of body type and weight loss, it will be greatly dependent on what your goals are and what changes you are hoping to achieve with your body. Losing weight for each body type can be achieved through adjustments in diets and exercise.

Those who have an ectomorph body type generally have an inability to gain muscle mass. So, in many cases, their goal may not be to lose weight per se. However, all body types can become overweight and may, at times, find it necessary to drop a few pounds. For example, if someone with an ectomorph body type develops hypothyroidism or hormonal irregularities, they may gain weight if they continue their eat anything and everything lifestyle. In these cases, they can work on weight or fat loss by doing resistance training and focusing on strength-building workouts. Remember earlier when we mentioned that muscle helps with losing weight or fat in the body? Well, by building muscle in an ectomorph body type, you will be able to reduce the fat in your body and overall increase your health. When it comes to the kitchen, those with an ectomorph body type can eat healthy fats, up to 30g of protein per meal, and have good quality and healthy carbs (Sims, 2016). If you are someone who particularly enjoys snacking, it may be best for you to adjust your meals depending on when you have a snack and when you work out. If you are going to work out early in the day, have a snack after breakfast, but if you're not working out, you can remove the snack entirely. Additionally, if you are having a late snack, you can opt to have a lighter dinner. This will help you meet your weight loss and fat loss goals for an ectomorph body type.

In most cases, those with an ectomorph body type tend to do well with carbohydrates that come from healthy sources. Fruit, veggies, and fiber-rich foods are the way to go.

People who have an endomorph body type may feel like they are really the ones who need to lose weight because they are the ones who generally have a rounder body type, especially around the midsection. Despite knowing that this is your body type and the one you have been born with, weight loss doesn't have to feel like an unreachable goal. As an endomorph, the goal is consistency. Exercise and healthy eating are the fundamentals to losing the weight that seems so easy to find you but so difficult to lose. High-intensity training and cross fit, which are a combination of cardio and strength training, are both great ways of losing weight. This, coupled with eating a high-fat and high-protein diet, is considered the optimal way for an endomorph to lose weight. This is because endomorphs tend to be much more sensitive to insulin spikes from carbohydrates, and those spikes can contribute to metabolic resistance. Consuming a high-fat and high-protein diet will minimize your cravings for carbs which have the ability to quickly push your insulin levels up. The most important thing in the case of having an endomorph body type is to build up a steady weight loss routine in both exercises and in your eating habits.

These sources of fats and proteins for a healthy endomorph diet can come from nuts, olive oils, beef, egg yolk, fish, and a wide variety of dairy products such as cheeses.

Those with a mesomorph body type find it easy to do sports that require speed and strength. Although they tend to lose and gain weight fast, there are things that those with this body type can do to optimize their weight loss. They tend to build muscle mass a lot faster, so endurance training and high-intensity interval training are great for them to quickly build up their muscle mass. Those with a mesomorph body type can eat high-quality fats and good carbs. Protein intake will not only prove to be beneficial to muscle gain, but if the person hopes to achieve weight loss instead of fat loss, they may not notice any change in the number on the scale because they may be building muscle at a higher rate than they are losing fat.

If someone with a mesomorph body type tends to find themself gaining weight (because, just like losing weight, it is easy to do), they may need to adjust their exercise focus to include more cardio.

Finding Your Body Type

Once you figure out what your body type is, one of two things can happen: you can fret that you don't have the body type you were hoping for, or you can take this knowledge and use the working hacks that are known to help with weight loss in these specific body types.

So how can you identify what body type you have?

Answer the questions below, and this will help you determine what your body type is (Catudal & Colino, 2019):

1. What is your shoulder-to-hip ratio?

A. My shoulders seem closer together than my hips.

B. My hips and shoulders appear to be the same width.

C. My hips are narrower than my shoulders.

2. If you had to analyze your body objectively in the mirror, what stands out and is more prominent in your body?

A. My bones are my most notable feature.

B. I have defined muscles.

C. I have more body fat than bone or muscle.

3. If you wrap your middle finger and thumb around your wrist...

A. the thumb and finger overlap.

B. the thumb and finger barely touch.

C. there is a gap between the thumb and finger.

4. What best describes your history in terms of the way your body looks and feels?

A. I have a hard time gaining muscle.

B. If I put my mind to it, gaining or losing weight is not too difficult.

C. I seem to gain weight easily, and it can take forever to lose weight.

5. What would you say you looked most like as a teenager?

A. Thin and lanky.

B. Strong and firm.

C. Soft and smooth.

Based on your answers to the previous questions, you can determine if you have an endomorph, ectomorph, or mesomorph body type. If your answers are predominantly made up of a's, you most likely have an ectomorph body type. If your answers are predominantly made of b's, you have a mesomorph body type. And finally, if you notice that c's seem to be your answers, then you probably have an endomorph body type.

Remember, don't be dismayed by the body type you may have. Instead, think of it as having insider info and a hack of knowing exactly what you need to do to lose weight.

Now that we have a baseline of what macros are and what the different body types are, we are going to look at how you can count and adjust your macros that will be perfect for your weight loss needs.

4

CALCULATING AND ADJUSTING MACROS

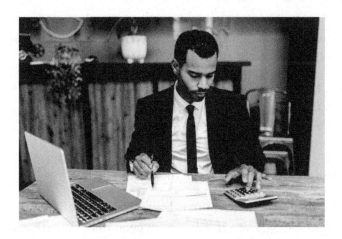

Knowing how our body works and processes energy is easy enough to understand, but it becomes slightly trickier when you put this knowledge into practice. It is all great if you know what macros are and what your body type is, but in this chapter, we are going to take what we know and what we have learned, and we are going to put it into practice in our lives.

A combination of macro counting and understanding how our body responds to these macros are some of the most important factors in reaching our weight loss goals. Once you understand how to calculate the macros you are meant to take in each day, you have a personalized dietary solution that will help you shed the pounds. Additionally, our body changes with each new phase of life that we enter, and as we enter each new phase, we then need to adjust our macros too. With this adjustment comes knowing and understanding when to change and adjust your macro intake.

In a world where everything is always balanced and both sides of the equation need to level out, calories have become an important part, not just in our bodies, but in terms of the energy input and expenditure that occurs. When you think about heat, one form of energy is used to create or give off heat energy. Energy isn't created but is rather converted, and this fundamental scientific equivalent, or equilibrium, is the fundamental concept that is used when we understand our consumption and use of calories as energy.

Basically, as much as we would like to think that calories are evil little creatures that make our clothes smaller, it is a unit of energy. It is the energy that we take in and use throughout our day.

Calculating Your Caloric Needs for Weight Loss

I am sure that at some point in our lives, we have all gone part of a day without eating, even if it has only been once. Whether it was a fast for religious purposes, fasting for diagnostic purposes whereby you would need to have blood work taken on an empty stomach, or not eating because you were just so caught up in a busy day that you didn't have a chance to eat, I can almost guarantee that about halfway through the day, you were probably feeling lethargic and like you were running on pure adrenaline more than actual energy. This is because our bodies aren't accustomed to going without food for long. Because we eat and drink our energy, unless we have trained our body to endure fasting, we need to consume food or nutrients to sustain not only the functions we carry out in the day but also for our bodies to run smoothly.

Let me give you a breakdown of what we would use energy for in a day. When we are doing absolutely nothing, I mean nothing at all, not even watching TV, or when we are sleeping, our body is using energy. As previously mentioned, our body uses energy when we are breathing, for our body to distribute oxygen into our cells, for our blood to move around our body, and for our heart to actively pump that blood (remember that there is not a single moment in our life where our hearts stop beating), and we use energy to digest foods and liquids that are in our bodies. When we do unconscious things, such as scratching an itch on our shoulder, yawning, laughing, or tapping our foot, we are also burning calories. And this is often done before we even get out of the bed in the morning.

Then we burn energy when we are awake, and we are walking from room to room. If you work at a desk job, you burn energy when your fingers are moving along the keyboard and typing. If your job is to carry letters from one floor to the next in an office building, you are also actively burning energy. If you work out, you then add to the energy that you are using.

And then, going even one step further, our brains need to function too. Every thought we have, and problem we actively try to solve uses some form of energy, even though it may not be as much as running laps on a track.

With all these calories that you are burning on a normal day, this is the reason why you would feel horrible and weak when you haven't eaten anything, or you missed a meal.

So how do you know how many calories you should be consuming, how do you know how many calories you need, and what is this information based on?

The number of calories you would need each day depends on a variety of factors such as your height, your weight, and whether you lead a sedentary or active lifestyle. If we look at balance and weight maintenance, we will need to consume as many calories as we burn each day. The calories that you burn at rest are known as your basal metabolic rate (BMR). This is the number of calories you burn by doing absolutely nothing, as mentioned above.

Here are three equations that can be used to calculate your BMR, each of which is different for men and for women (Calorie Calculator, n.d.):

Mifflin-St Jeor Equation:

For men is 10W + 6.25H - 5A + 5

For women is 10W + 6.25H - 5A - 161

Revised Harris-Benedict Equation:

For men is 13.397W + 4.799H - 5.677A + 88.362

For women is 9.247W + 3.098H - 4.330A + 447.593

Katch-McArdle Formula:

BMR = 370 + 21.6(1 - F)W

In each of these equations, W is your body weight in kgs, H is your height in cm, A is age, and F is your body fat percentage.

How Many Calories Do You Need?

One of the most simple and straightforward ways of understanding weight loss is to consume fewer calories than you burn at rest. This means that your calorie consumption needs to be less than the number you obtained from any of the above equations. However, the thing about calories is that it is not as simple as consuming fewer calories to lose weight; you need to consume a specific number of calories to maintain a healthy balance. When you consume too few calories, you end up putting your body in a state of starvation where it holds calorie stores instead of burning calories.

With one pound equating to around 3,500 calories, you would need to remove 3,500 calories from your diet. Realistically, this cannot be done in one try or in one day. However, you can work on a weekly basis, depending on your goals and the rate at which you are hoping to lose weight. So, you could cut down your weekly calorie intake by 3,500 calories, and you would lose one pound of weight in that week.

For example, when I began my weight loss journey, my BMR was about 1,300 calories. This was how many calories my body burns at rest each day. When I added in my activity, my Total Daily Energy Expenditure (which we will address shortly) was right around 1,700 calories. If I wanted to lose one pound immediately, I would have needed to consume zero calories for about two days just to lose one pound of weight. However, if I had cut out about 500 calories a day, my daily consumption to lose weight would have been 1,200 calories per day, and I would have lost one pound in a week.

I know this may seem hard to do, especially when you think about how little you would need to eat to consume 1,200 calories a day; however, when you consider that not all calories are created equally, this makes it easier to understand the logic and nutrition that comes with weight loss and your calorie intake.

For example, as a rough estimate, when you consider that a 100g chocolate chip cookie has about the same number of calories as almost nine 100g apples, it becomes clear to see that not all calories are the same. Now, let me pose the instance of eating 1,200 calories a day for weight loss. Many people argue that 1,200 calories doesn't seem like a lot or enough to sustain you. However, if you are filling those calories with nutritious foods, you can actually be sustained with only 800 calories, and still lose weight in a healthy way (Abet, 2019).

Here is an example of what I would typically eat in a day (I am an ectomorph with severe thyroid struggles, so while my body looked more like an endomorph at the time, I needed to eat like an ectomorph to see weight loss results):

Breakfast: 4 oz. apple, 2 slices of whole grain toast, 1 tbsp. butter, coffee with monk fruit sweetener.

Lunch: 4 oz. Ground Sirloin, 4 oz. Riced Cauliflower, 4 oz. sauteed red onions, 4 oz. sauteed mushrooms, ¼ cup of 1% cottage cheese, small, sweet potato, 4 oz. strawberries, spinach salad with sliced peppers and balsamic vinegar for dressing. I mix the ground sirloin with the sauteed vegetables and make a salad with the raw vegetables.

Snack: 12 mini peppers

Dinner: 4 oz. Pork Loin, 4 oz. sauerkraut, 4 oz. green beans, 4 oz. cantaloupe, 1 slice of whole wheat bread.

The macronutrient breakdown for this day was approximately: 56% carbs, 25% proteins, and 19% fats, with a total of around 1,235 calories. It may not fit exactly into the macro ratios for an ectomorph, but it's very close, and it includes a variety of nutritious and very filling foods.

Since you have a daily allotted number of calories to consume, it would be wise to consume foods that keep you fuller for longer, rather than taking in one calorie-dense snack and being hungry and cranky for the rest of the day. So, if you are consuming 1,200 calories a day for weight loss, you would probably want to avoid things like chocolate chip cookies because a couple ounces of cookies won't fill you up, but it will take up a large portion of your allotted calories for the day. This being said, the beauty of counting macros is that you are able to eat that chocolate chip cookie or even a piece of cake if it fits your macros.

I recommend you follow the 80/20 principal, where 80% of your macros come from whole foods that are healthy, but the other 20%

can be made up of indulgences. This is perfect if you are going to an event, and you know will have tempting foods. Using the 80/20 principal, considering 21 meals each week, that would allow you 4 indulgences each week! When I indulge, I still try and do my best to stay within my daily macro allowance. I recommend you choose a menu that you've already tried, and you know fits your macros, then eliminate foods to replace with your indulgence of choice. Let's look at the previous 1,200-calorie example and see how I would adapt that menu so I could indulge in a piece of cake at a party that afternoon.

Breakfast: 4 oz. apple

Lunch: 4 oz. Ground Sirloin, 4 oz. Riced Cauliflower, 4 oz. sauteed red onions, 4 oz. sauteed mushrooms, ¼ cup of 1% cottage cheese, 4 oz. strawberries, spinach salad with sliced peppers and balsamic vinegar for dressing. I mix the ground sirloin with the sauteed vegetables and make a salad with the raw vegetables.

Snack: 1 piece of cake with icing at a party

Dinner: 4 oz. Pork Loin, 4 oz. sauerkraut, 4 oz. green beans, 4 oz. cantaloupe, 1 slice of whole wheat bread.

The macronutrient breakdown for this day was approximately: 56% carbs, 25% proteins, and 19% fats, with a total of around 1,235 calories. Again, it may not fit exactly into the macro breakdown, but it's very close. In order to enjoy a guilt free indulgence later that day, I eliminated the toast and butter from breakfast, and I eliminated the sweet potato from lunch. I kept the most nutrient dense fruits and vegetables for the most part to make this work for my health goals. Shifting your macros around is simple if you use an app that breaks your foods down into macros and calories.

How to Calculate Your Macro Needs

Counting your macro consumption provides you with parameters in which you can still enjoy a seemingly endless variety of foods while still losing weight and staying healthy. You can eat everything you want, provided it is within the confines of your macro consumption. But how do you calculate the exact number of macros that you need to consume daily, while factoring in your BMR, whether you do any physical activities during the day, and your body type?

Your BMR is calculated as your resting energy expenditure, as previously mentioned. This is counted when you are doing absolutely nothing. However, when you factor in that most people do some sort of physical exercise, whether it is walking, mild exercising, or extreme workouts, the number of calories you burn is even greater. This is known as your total daily energy expenditure (TDEE), whereby you factor in how many calories you burn at rest, including the calories burned during physical activity. The number of calories you burn during a workout can be calculated depending on a few factors, such as whether you lead a sedentary lifestyle, a moderately active lifestyle, or a very active lifestyle. In each case, when you complete the above-mentioned formulas to obtain your BMR, particularly in the Mifflin-St Jeor formula, you will include an additional step to calculate your TDEE.

Mifflin-St Jeor Equation:

For men it is $10W + 6.25H - 5A + 5$

For women it is $10W + 6.25H - 5A - 161$

If you lead a sedentary lifestyle, you will multiply the answer on the above-mentioned formula by 1.2, by 1.55 if you lead a moderately active lifestyle, and by 1.735 if you lead a very active lifestyle (Kallmyer, 2021).

Once you have this number in hand, which is unique to you and your body's dimensions, you can then begin working out how many macros you need to consume. To lose weight consistently, you need to be in a calorie deficit, consuming less than what you are taking in. While the general rule of thumb is to decrease your calorie intake by 500 calories, this is just a general estimation and doesn't consider your body type and the specifics of your body's structure. To get a more customized estimation of how many calories you should cut out each day to lose weight is to reduce your calorie intake by 20%. This means that whatever number you get in the TDEE calculation, you would subtract 20% from that number, and that's the number of calories you would consume each day for weight loss. This calculation would mean someone with a TDEE of 1,700 would lower their daily calorie intake by 440 calories. It may take a little longer to drop those extra pounds, but the best diet is the one you can stick to. If going by the 20% reduction helps keep your hunger at bay, you are much more likely to reach your goals. You must find what works for you.

But still, this equation is flawed in terms of personalization. There can be two people who have the exact same number of TDEE. One person can be heavier and maybe even obese, but they can also be extremely short, and another can be tall and lean. The number of calories that each person consumes would mathematically be the same; however, the person who is obese and has an endomorph body type is not recommended to consume the same macro ratios as the ectomorph body type. While the number of calories they should consume is the same in terms of numbers, the person who is obese or overweight with an endomorph body type would need to eat substantially fewer macronutrients that fall under the category of carbs, than the person with the ectomorph body type. This is why counting macros work so well!

According to Ted Kallmyer (2021) and Amanda Capritto (2022), there are ways to calculate exactly how many fats, carbs, and protein you need to consume, depending on your goals.

There is a general ratio that you can expect to consume in terms of how many macros you need. For the most part, your ration should be made up of between 45% to 60% carbohydrates, 20% to 35% fats, and the rest of the remaining percentage should come from your protein consumption. But this general rule of thumb is not great, and all it does is provide you with a general range instead of exact percentages according to your own body type and weight.

Here are some ways that you can calculate your macro needs exactly, according to your body's needs:

- Protein—depending on your body type and goals, your protein requirements will differ. If you engage in heavy weightlifting, you will need to consume one gram of protein per pound of your body weight. This is because your body needs proteins for repairing and building muscle.

If you are hoping to maintain your weight and you are doing moderate training, you would need to consume about 0.825g of protein for every pound of body weight.

If you are hoping to lose weight and reduce body fat, you would need to consume about 0.65g of protein per pound of body weight.

So, for example, if you weigh 152 pounds and you are doing moderate exercises, you will calculate how many grams of protein you would need through this equation: 152 x 0.825. This would mean that you would need to consume about 125g of protein daily.

- Fat—When it comes to fat, our bodies actually need it to survive. In doing so, having the correct amount is of paramount importance. Falling in the range of 20% to 35%, your diet does seem to require a decent amount of fat. But once again, this will depend on your goals and the type of diet you are on. For weight loss, perhaps let us use the example of 25% of your macros being made up of fat. In this case, to measure how many grams of fat you need to consume, you would need to use your TDEE calories as a rule of thumb. Let us say, for example, that your TDEE calories are 2,500. If your fats need to make up 25%, you can multiply your TDEE calories by 25% (2,500 x 0.25 = 625). This means that 625 of your daily calories would need to come from a fat source. Because we know that every gram of fat has 9 calories, we can divide 625 by 9, and that is how many grams of fat you would need each day (625 ÷ 9 = 69 g).

- Carbs—Carbohydrates are the fuel that keeps our bodies running optimally. When you consume carbs, you give your body the energy it needs to survive. Just in the same way that you measure your fat, you are going to use your TDEE calories to calculate what ratio of your macros should be made up of carbs. Through simple subtraction and knowing how many calories exist in a gram of protein, fat, and carbs, you can easily calculate just how much carbs you will need to consume in a day. If your protein consumption is 125g, this means 500 calories of your daily 2,500 calorie intake belongs to protein (125g x 4 calories per gram of protein). In terms of fat, 69g means that 625 calories are allocated to this macro, and therefore the remainder would be allocated to the carbs you should be consuming. To calculate this, it would be: 2,500 - (625 + 500) = 1,375 of your calories should come from carbs. Further, you could work out the grams by dividing the 1,375 by 4 (which is the number of calories per gram for carbs), and this gives you about 344g of carbs that you need to consume.

Therefore, the macronutrient ratio for someone who has a TDEE of 2,500 calories would need to consume 125g of protein, 69g of fat, and 344 g of carbs.

One thing that is extremely important to remember during your macro counting journey is that it takes dedication. Every single thing that you consume has specific nutritional information. You will rarely consume something that is only protein, only fat, or only a carb. Instead, its complex composition is made up of a variety of nutrients.

For example, one serving of a banana has about one gram of protein, 28g of carbs, and three grams of fiber (Harvard School of Public Health, 2018). This means that when you eat a banana, you need to consider how much it contributes to each of your daily macro consumption. Just in the same way, a 100g steak will have about 35g of protein and about 10g of fat. You cannot eat a 100g steak and assume that it is going to count entirely toward your protein intake. Instead, you need to be conscious and aware of the macronutrients in each item of food that you are consuming.

Macros for Your Body Type

Once you determine your TDEE, you also need to consider that each person's body type is different. How would you know with your endomorph body type how much fat is too much? How would you know if you are lacking protein with your ectomorph body type?

Based on the calculations above, you can split your macro intake for each body type according to the following percentages (Savino, 2020):

- In general, ectomorph body types need around 55% of the macros to come from carbs, 25% to come from protein, and 20% to come from fats.
- Endomorph body types generally require their macros to come from 25% carbs, 35% proteins, and 40% fats.
- The mesomorph body type requires about 40% carbs, 30% proteins, and 30% fats.

Having this blueprint in hand makes it easier to identify exactly what you need to eat in a way that is optimized for you. I know that it can seem to be a lot of work, which is why to start with, I strongly recommend using a macros app now that you know the ratios for your personal body type. Before you know it, you will be counting macros with one eye closed, and you know exactly what it is you are putting in your body.

Converting Your Own Calories Into Macro Grams

Now that you have an understanding of how your calories and macros work, you can now apply this to your life in a practical way. Now is the time to bring out the mathematician in yourself, and it is time to calculate what exactly you need to be consuming.

Using the preceding calculations under the How to Calculate Your Macro Needs section, you can work out the exact ratio of macronutrients that you would need to lose, gain, or maintain the weight that also takes into account the type of exercise you are doing.

The thing about counting macros to lose weight is that it is a hack that you have the power to use to actually shed the pounds. All the diets that have never worked before can be thrown out the window when you have the knowledge of counting macros.

Do you want to know what is the best part about counting macros? Once you lose the weight and you reach your goal and target weight, you can easily adjust the macros you should be consuming to maintain your weight. This keeps you healthy and happy!

In the next chapter, we are going to take a deeper dive into how to keep track of your macros and how to make it a task that is part of your daily life, instead of something that is difficult or that feels like an effort and an annoyance. Instead of feeling like a job, it becomes a habit, and eventually, you won't even realize you're doing it.

5

HOW TO TRACK MACROS

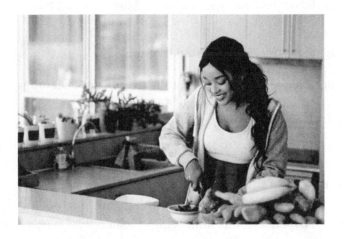

Remember that tracking macros helps make sure you are eating the right ratios of essential nutrients and helps you control your weight. I can assure you that tracking macros isn't that hard, and it isn't as toilsome as you might expect. What I have come to learn on my weight loss journey is that if you are willing to put in the work to lose weight and build a healthier lifestyle, chances are you are fully prepared to use a kitchen scale to weigh out your food, or do the math required to determine the macros in your favorite casserole.

And if you are willing to do that, you can take comfort in knowing that steps like these are just what it takes to reach your goals.

Once you understand the underlying principles of what macros are and how they interact with our body, once you understand what the value of a macro is, everything else seems to fall into place. Counting your macros becomes easier and more transparent, and in the next chapter, we delve deeper into how you can track macros in a more simplified way through meal planning. But aside from understanding the science behind it, we also live in technology's prime time. There is an app for everything. . . including counting macros. This not only makes it easy to do, but it also means that, for the most part, you don't have to be calculating everything you eat. Instead, you have a handy app that does it for you.

So let us delve into counting macros and how this can be easily done.

How to Track Your Macros Step by Step

In earlier chapters, we have established an understanding of what macros are and why our bodies need them. We have also come to appreciate why our bodies need macronutrients in the correct ratios and why this, in turn, promotes weight loss, assists in healthy weight gain, or helps you maintain a healthy weight. From this, we see the importance of nutrient tracking not only in maintaining a healthy weight but also in obtaining everything that our body *needs*. You know when you are uncomfortable, bloated, and just not feeling great after a meal? You're feeling tired and cranky, and you just don't know why? Most likely, your body hasn't gotten what it needs, it is unhappy, and it must work twice or three times harder to accommodate what you have fed into it. When you understand the science behind macros, you realize that fundamentally, you begin giving your body not just what it craves but what it needs. You do it in a healthy way that makes your body thank you for what you've eaten rather than making you feel miserable.

This is how you can count your macros in three easy steps:

Step 1: Understand Your Macros

The first step in beginning your macro tracking journey is what we have been doing in this book: First, you build an understanding of what macros are. Then you use this knowledge to determine your caloric needs and your body type. The knowledge behind macros, coupled with firm goals in place, gives you a personalized method of using macros for your own personal benefit.

When you establish your goals, you need to decide on the amount of weight you would like to lose, and determine the timeframe needed to lose that weight in a healthy way.

Once you have your goal firmly in mind, you can then decipher how many grams of carbs, proteins, and fats you need to reach your goal based on your body type. And finally, once you are equipped with this knowledge, you have the weight loss/muscle gain/weight mainte-nance blueprint that needs to be put into practice for you to meet your goals.

Step 2: Get the Right Tools

There are a few tools that you *need* when you begin tracking your macros. The good news is that all the tools you need are easily acces-sible and will make the entire process that much easier.

The first tool you need comes from within you, and that is your *why*. You need to know *why* you *want* to make a change. I know this seems like a straightforward want to have, but many people don't seem to realize they need to make a change in their lives until they receive a diagnosis, or they realize they can't play with their grandkids anymore, or they find themselves tired and unhappy with their phys-ical bodies. Having a why increases willpower and this is the best way I know to not only start but maintain your journey because, after all, that is what this is—a journey.

Next, you need some form of accountability. This, coupled with the actual tool that you will use to track your macros, will make your entire weight loss journey much more successful. There are countless tools in the form of applications, as we mentioned, that can help you track your macros. You see, when you actively start tracking your macros, you need to be accountable to the tool you are using, making sure that you input what you are eating. Now, the tool you use to track your macros could be a digital application, or it could be a good old-fashioned pen and paper. Whatever it is, it will help keep you on track. MyFitnessPal, Nutritionix Track, Cronometer, LoseIt!, LifeSum, or MyMacros+ are all great examples of macro counting applications available to you.

In many cases, people find accountability in the form of other people and in groups as opposed to accountability methods that don't include other people. Many mobile applications have an option that allows you to be a part of a greater community. Additionally, you have access to an endless database of food, which will make your macro-counting journey easier and more enjoyable.

The most important physical tool you need to get started is a digital kitchen scale. When you begin counting macros, you absolutely must weigh out your portions for proper macro counting. At first, most people are unable to accurately determine how many grams or ounces a given food weighs, and knowing this is the basis for counting macros. When going out to restaurants, you can either carry along a pocket scale, or you can estimate and count the meal as part of your 20% if you are following the 80/20 principle.

Step 3: Log Your Daily Intake

This is the step where you are actually doing the work. For every other part of these three steps, you are just gathering the tools and making sure you are motivated to begin. Here is where you begin.

You need to care enough about your weight loss journey to put effort into counting your macros and tracking them each day. No one is with you as much as you are with yourself, and therefore only you can keep track of what you are putting into your body. The tools you have can't work effectively unless you actually put them to use. Now, this is the part that may seem tedious and time-consuming because you do need to record every single thing that you put into your mouth. A lot of the times, people forget that they also need to count and take into consideration what they drink. Without tracking, we can inadvertently drink our calories and macronutrients.

Think about it this way, if you have a chocolate milkshake with a chicken salad, you may not be eating your calories, or you may not be consuming as many calories as you would be if you were eating a slice of pizza, but you cannot forget about the calories in your drink. In your chocolate milkshake alone, you will find a lot of each of your macronutrients, but you will also be consuming more than 300 calories in your drink alone. In such cases, you could have possibly eaten a delicious slice of pizza along with a glass of water. Much in the same way as someone may prefer drinking a protein shake, while they may understand it contributes to their protein count for the day, it may slip their mind that it adds to their calories, and instead of being in a calorie deficit to lose weight, they find themselves maintaining or gaining weight.

One thing that macro tracking will help you do, is it will make you more conscious and aware of your portion control. Initially, when you begin your tracking and weight loss journey, you may become slightly annoyed by the fact that you must weigh everything and be conscious of the serving size you are consuming. Thankfully, almost everything you eat has a portion control recommendation along with a recommended serving size. In most cases, macro tracking applications will be able to keep track of the nutritional value of the serving size you have eaten. If you are making a meal from scratch, all you need to do is keep track of the weight of each ingredient you include in the meal, record it in your macro tracking app, and once the meal is cooked, you can measure the serving you are consuming, and the app will tell you exactly what the calories are in that meal along with the macronutrient contents.

While this may seem like work initially because you do have to measure your portions, eventually, you become accustomed to how much you eat, and you automatically begin practicing portion control. It becomes easier to stop yourself from overeating and therefore sticking to your macronutrient intake each day. Eventually, you won't even need the kitchen scale, and you will have a great understanding of how much food should be on your plate for you to meet your macro goals.

In addition to drinks, something else that we also tend to forget to count are our snacks and added toppings. Whether it is those few chips you took from your child's snack, the ketchup you added to your fries, the salad dressing, or even the olive oil that you used when cooking your meal, always make sure you record these often-forgotten items. Additionally, I have found that it is always great to record your meals and snacks immediately so that you don't give yourself an opportunity to forget.

And finally, we have already established that using a mobile app takes a lot of the guesswork out of recording your daily meals. It is important, however, that you remain as accurate as possible. This means that you should also include specific brands or scan the barcodes of any food items where possible because this will account for any variation between brands (Slabaugh, 2017).

An example of macro tracking would mean that you count the proteins, carbs, and fats in your two scrambled eggs that were made in a teaspoon of butter. Your tracker will tell you the value of each macronutrient in this meal, including the macros in your coffee that had milk and sweetener in it. Macro tracking will do the same for the snacks, lunch, and dinner you have, giving you your total daily consumption, which can then be easily measured up to your daily macro allowance. Once you have this down to a tee, it shouldn't take you more than five minutes before each meal to record your macros.

Also, recording your macros before your meal reduces the chances of you going back and having a second serving. And finally, because humans are creatures of habit, you will eventually fall into a routine of repeating certain dishes, especially ones that are your favorites. This will make recording your nutrients much simpler. But we will take a closer look at meal prep in the next chapter.

Adjusting Your Macros

Like everything else in your life, as soon as you hit your stride and you have found the perfect way to track your macros, you may find that you have lost weight, and then you will need to make some adjustments. The great thing is that once you start counting your macros, you never have to start from scratch, but you rather just need to adjust your macros according to the changes in your body and your new goals.

In many cases, your goals may not change immediately. Perhaps you hoped to lose 10 pounds, but you have only lost 6 pounds. You can adjust your macro intake according to your new goal, which is no longer to lose 10 pounds but to lose 4 pounds. Just in the same way, if you had reached your goal, you may decide that you now want to build muscle mass or you want to maintain your weight. These are the new goals you are hoping to achieve, and you can adjust your macros accordingly.

Here are some tips that you can keep in mind when you are adjusting your macros:

- Always reassess your goals: As mentioned before, you will need to adjust your goals according to the weight loss you experience, especially if you experience major weight loss.
- Do an assessment of your progress: You know when you start a beginner's workout, you first need to master that workout before you move on to the next one? Well, the same thing goes for counting your macros. If you are unable to stick to

and maintain your macro intake, your water intake, a fitness regiment, and resting between workouts, then you may not be able to adjust your macros just yet. In stages, it is always better to master the first before you move on to the second.

- Keep track of your accomplishments: You can't adjust your macros with every pound or ounce that you lose. This is neither beneficial nor helpful. Give yourself realistic milestones and goals to work toward. Use measurements, progress pictures, and the scale as a way of assessing how much you have accomplished and if you have the need to adjust your macros (Field, 2022).

It is also important to remember that with diet comes fitness and exercise. In the calculations we did in the previous chapter, we adjusted the number according to the level of fitness you may have, whether that was a sedentary lifestyle, a moderately active lifestyle, or an active lifestyle. The more you work out and exercise, the stronger you will get and the more you will be able to do.

There is a general rule of thumb you can follow depending on the type of training you are doing and how this aligns with your goals. If you are hoping to consume specific macros while you are weight training, there are important factors to consider. Weight training and weight loss aren't two separate entities and usually work hand in hand with each other. However, for weight loss purposes, you will be consuming a calorie deficit. This deficit is likely to cause you to lose muscle mass, and if you are weight training, this is obviously something you are going to try to avoid. The best way to avoid this or mitigate this is to increase your protein consumption which not only aids in muscle recovery but also prevents you from losing too much of your muscle mass in your weight loss journey (Collova, 2019).

When it comes to cardio training, this depends more on your body type than it does on the type of macros you're eating. While ectomorphs typically need to load up on carbs before they do cardio, endomorphs typically need more fat.

While it is not unheard of or impossible to adjust your macronutrient ratio on a daily basis, especially to factor in things like the type of workouts you are going to be doing, it is not something that is needed. I have come to find that micromanaging your food intake and the way you eat can quickly begin to feel like a chore rather than something that is just part of your lifestyle. I have found that your enjoyment comes with the routine of having figured out what worked best for you and letting it stick or settle in for a little while before changing it up. But remember that this is all about balance; it is about enjoying what you eat while still staying healthy. So let the small stuff slide, and you will find yourself happier because your comeback will be so much greater. After all, we all face setbacks, but that doesn't mean that we stop the entire process and throw away all the progress we have made just because we didn't record the one candy bar we ate without tracking it.

Common Macro Counting Mistakes to Avoid

With all great plans and systems in place come the mistakes that people make when they use these plans, and counting macros is no different. Counting your macros to lose weight is not something that is fool-proof, and people tend to make mistakes when doing so. These are some of the common mistakes people make when counting macros to lose weight (Brueseke, 2018):

- Many people get confused that calories and macros are not the same. In some cases, there may be days when you consume too much of one of your macros, and many people wonder if they should still be eating the same amount of the other two macros. For weight loss purposes, eating too much of one macro will mean that you would need to reduce your consumption of the other two macros because to achieve weight loss, you need to be in a calorie deficit.
- This is not an overnight thing. Many people make the mistake of giving up too soon because they don't see results.

Now, I know results are what keep us motivated. But if you decide to pursue macro counting as a method of weight loss, it is something that you are going to need to stay committed to, and it is not something that is going to yield results immediately.

- We've already discussed this previously, but a common mistake that people make is that they try to adjust their macros on a daily or weekly basis. You don't need to adjust your macros for every pound that you lose, but instead, Brueseke (2018) states that if you are continuously seeing results, you can stick with your current macro ratio. The only time you may need to consider adjusting your macros is if you reach a plateau and, for two weeks or more, you don't see any changes in your body.

- Another common mistake is not consuming enough water. At a molecular level, consuming more protein increases the amount of nitrogen in our bodies, and this nitrogen needs to be flushed out with water through our urine. If it isn't flushed out, it can cause constipation. This means that more protein, if not consumed with water, can easily lead to constipation, and many people make the mistake of not increasing their water intake when they up their protein macros.

- We know that measuring your food is an important part of tracking macros, but in many cases, the macro composition of foods may change after they are cooked. In fact, when cooked, meat can lose up to a quarter of its weight (Warshaw, 2014). For that reason, when you are weighing meat, be sure to be consistent with weighing your meat cooked.

- Another mistake that people make is that they eyeball their serving sizes, and they usually get their estimates wrong. You do need to get in the visual habit of seeing your general serving sizes before you begin eyeballing them. I can guarantee you that, at first, you will wrongly consume certain amounts of food if you don't weigh them because eyeballing weight is tricky to do.

Tools and Apps for Counting Macros

I think one of the most underrated benefits of counting macros, aside from the obvious weight loss and health benefits that you will experience, is that you don't have to do it by yourself. The counting, the tracking, the remembering—none of it must be done in your mind and instead, there are countless applications that do the work for you.

These apps work on a database that, much like artificial intelligence, is always developing and enhancing itself. Each new food item and new food combination that is added to each application is recorded and can then be reused and readjusted according to the amount and weight of the food you are eating. These apps not only track the macronutrients you are consuming, but they also track and monitor your calorie intake, making sure that you aren't taking in too many calories, especially if you are trying to lose weight.

But even beyond tracking, many of these apps work in a way that also prompts you to record how you are feeling after each meal and can then devise a tally of how certain foods actually make you feel. This will obviously impact and influence how often you choose to consume that food again in the future.

Some of the most popular apps that you could choose from include MyFitnessPal, Nutritionix Track, Cronometer, LoseIt!, LifeSum, or MyMacros+.

Creating Your Action Plan

Now, it is time for you to start your plan toward counting macros for weight loss. It starts with having your calculations in place. Once you know exactly how much you are meant to consume, you can then begin finding an app that works for you. This may take a small trial period because you may prefer an app that has some features as opposed to those that don't have this particular feature. You may find an application that has multiple features that you don't use, so try a different one. Whatever it is, finding the best fit for you is of utmost importance.

Then you need to make the time commitment to tracking your macros. Remember, this isn't going to start off as a walk in the park. If you know that you are going on a breakfast date with friends and you have a birthday dinner on the same day, it either isn't the best day to start, or it is going to be a day that is going to require some planning so that you can adjust what you eat.

Finally, if you can get others involved in this journey, it will make the entire experience that much easier. Remember, walking a long journey alone is harder than if you have company. Finding a community will make tracking your macros that much easier.

In the next chapter, we are going to delve into something that is not only beneficial in tracking your macros, but that also makes tracking that much easier—meal planning. During meal planning and meal prep, you put all the intellectual work behind counting macros into one day, and you get to enjoy each meal with ease thereafter. Because of this prep, you may find yourself having a more enjoyable experience counting your macros in the days to come because half the job has already been done when you were prepping your meals.

6

MEAL PLANNING AND PREPPING

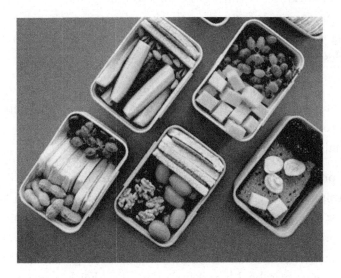

This has to be, without a doubt, one of my favorite parts about counting macros and about being on this weight loss journey with this particular method. If you're anything like me, you fawn over the organizational posts that come across your social media feed. You look on in admiration as meals are prepared in advance, and you see them grabbing their lunch with no fuss, no calculations done in the background, and no numbers or scales while they enjoy their meal. This is because meal prep helps isolate the hard work of counting your macros to one day so that every other day, you get to enjoy ease and convenience. Now if you ask me, one day of hard work behind the kitchen scale and with a calculator seems like a fair and easy trade for grab-and-go meals, plus promised weight loss. Not only that but having food always ready to eat means that even at your hungriest moment, you won't need to buy takeout or eat any of the unhealthy stuff that you should actively avoid.

As important as prepping our meals are, part of meal planning also involves when you eat. This combination of *what* and *when* gives you the best outcomes for the goals you are hoping to achieve. You see, if you are working out during the day, you are going to want to make your macros work for you so that you have enough energy to use during your workout and that you have enough protein to help your muscles repair after the workout.

I know it seems more complex, but once you get the hang of it, just like counting your macros, this all becomes easier and better. You learn your body, and what you put in your body gets used in the most optimal way.

Meal prep is probably a term that you're familiar with. In fact, you may think that it is something that has garnered a lot of popularity in the last few years. However, you might be surprised to know that meal prep and the trend surrounding meal prep grew in popularity between the 1980s and the 1990s. It seems many great trends tend to form as part of a health and fitness routine that has taken over the world. The same is true for meal prep, and in the 80's and 90's it was popular in many fitness magazines as a way of encouraging weight loss and building muscle (Khurshid, 2022).

But the reason why meal prep is so popular and has gained so much traction in modern society is because the benefits are insurmountable. People have tried and tested it, and they have found the benefits of meal prep. In fact, you will find that a lot of people who have tried meal prep have found it so beneficial that they are unlikely to go back to cooking meals each and every day.

Benefits of Preparing Meals Ahead of Time

One of the best and easiest ways of accommodating your macros in your meal planning is to use the following hack: By now, we have already established that having a macro tracking app is going to make your life substantially easier. But to make counting your macros and your ratios that much easier, especially for meal prep, you can start with a benchmark baseline of 4 to 6 ounces of protein, 4 to 6 ounces of fruit, or 100 calories of a starchy food, 4 to 6 ounces of non-starchy vegetables, and a couple of tablespoons of good, healthy fats. This is just a general rule of thumb, but it makes meal prep easier knowing that you have a balanced nutritional plan based on the protein, carbs, and fats that comprise your meal. You can then add variation to your meal by adjusting the proteins, fat, and carbs accordingly.

Allow me to delve deeper into some of the benefits you can experience if you choose to use this method of preparing food.

The first benefit is the one that has already been mentioned, and this is because it is the most obvious benefit and the most notable one. We all want extra time. We want to spend more time with our kids, our families, and our loved ones. While preparing meals in advance may not allow us to tack days and months into our lives, it does save us time each day because we don't have to prepare a meal from scratch. Yes, you are spending time one day a week preparing for the remainder of the week but think about the two hours you spend meal prepping in one day so that you can save an hour each day for the rest of the week. That is a fair trade to make.

Meal prepping will save you money! Think about these two scenarios: The first is that every day for a week, you cook a new evening meal. But the amount that you cook is slightly more than what your family can consume. This usually means that there are leftovers, but it is not enough to make an entire meal for a person. The food ends up staying at the back of the fridge, and it either ends up going bad, or you find yourself tossing it out because no one, including you, is willing to eat it. The second scenario is similar, but it applies more to raw ingredients. I am sure we have all had the experience where we bought fresh groceries and planned what we were going to make each day. Then, lo and behold, we got tired or busy. Rather than making the meal we planned, we ended up ordering takeout, and all the fresh foods went bad in our fridge. In both scenarios, you end up wasting food and you end up throwing your money away. Meal prep makes sure that all ingredients are used and portioned off so that there are no leftovers, everything is consumed, and no unnecessary foods are purchased.

Just in the same way, as previously mentioned, meal prep makes sure that there are always ready-to-eat meals in your home. This means less takeout, less junk, and a healthier lifestyle.

Think about a big Sunday lunch or Thanksgiving meal. When you dish the food onto your plate, even if you have been counting macros for a while and you know your general serving size, it is all too easy to go back for a second or put a little too much on your plate. And because you hate wasting, you make sure you finish everything on your plate. When you prep your meals in advance, you can better exercise portion control, and you lower the risk of overeating. Yes, you can officially say goodbye to being uncomfortably full and having to loosen your pants button because you have eaten too much.

Decision fatigue is one of the things that most people struggle with. Imagine if you didn't have to decide what to eat or what meal to prepare on a daily basis. That sounds like a dream, right? Well, meal prep does that because, in most cases, knowing you've prepared in advance means you don't have to worry about what you or your family are eating until the time comes to heat up your food.

Another obvious benefit is that when you prepare your meals, you have the power to make sure that every meal has all the macros that your body needs. This includes health, variation, and enjoyment. Also, to be honest, there is a unique sense contentment that comes with knowing what you are going to eat each day. If you're anything like me, it's like researching the menu at a restaurant you're heading to so that you know exactly what you're going to order.

Scientifically, meal prep has also been shown to have several benefits. From obesity prevention to contributing to your emotional well-being, it seems to pose multiple unseen benefits to people (Blanton, 2022).

Now that we know all the benefits that meal prep provides to us, you're probably wondering how to start. Well, let us get into the tips and tricks that you need for meal prep.

Meal Planning Strategies and Tips

Maybe one of the concerns you have about meal prep is that you may be unsettled by the idea of you or your family eating the same meal every day for a week. But that's not how it works. There are many ways to add variety to your meal prep, and one of the major benefits is that you never have to question, "What's for lunch/dinner?"

There are many ways to prepare meals that include variation. On the day that you do your shopping and your meal prep, you can plan for each day, or you can plan for the week. I have found that both meal preps for families and meal preps for an individual can include variation and repetition is not inevitable.

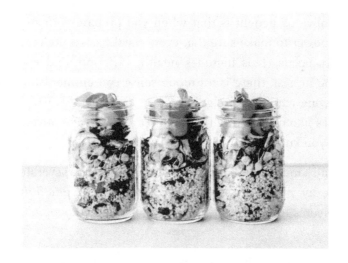

One way of getting around the repetition of foods is that you can plan a set menu and rotate on a weekly basis. There are a few ways of bringing consistent recipes into rotation. The first thing you can do is have about six of your favorite recipes that contain the exact amounts and ratios of your macronutrients. On your meal prep day, you can choose two of your six favorite meals and prepare those two meals for the week, alternating the meal you eat each day. This means that you won't be eating the same thing two days in a row. The following week, you can prepare your next two dishes, which will be different from the previous week, and so on and so forth. This gives you great variation while ensuring that you don't get tired of eating the same thing over and over again.

If you are preparing meals that fare quite well with freezing, you could work on a daily theme. This means that each day, you will be eating something different, and if you prepare enough of each meal, you could freeze your meals for the next week as well.

Beyond this, there are other ways to add variation to your meals. Something as simple as swapping out one macro each day for a different type can change your entire meal. If your meal prep includes avocado as a fat and brown rice as the carb, you could switch your protein and alternate steak on a Monday, chicken on a Tuesday, tuna on a Wednesday, and then you could go back to steak. Alternatively, you could also switch out the fat that you are eating and change out the avocado for some nuts or the rice for a healthy bread. When you think about the different variations, they seem endless.

Another tip that you could use when you are preparing your meals for the week, is that you can make a detailed shopping list that includes all the ingredients you need for each meal. This will help you make sure you don't forget ingredients, and it will also prevent you from buying snacks that shouldn't be on your list.

You may find that while you are meal prepping, half of the task is completed merely by chopping all your fruits and vegetables. You can save a lot of time just doing what I call power hour prep. When power hour prepping you simply chop and measure out all the vegetables you will be using for the upcoming week, so they are ready to cook when you get home. If you are preparing a meal that doesn't necessarily need to be cooked, such as a salad, then cutting and chopping is the most work you're going to be doing (aside from weighing your meals and recording the details onto the databases on your macro tracking app).

One thing I have found when shopping for my meal prep is that I am always able to save money with the two-for-one or the other specials that I find in the store. These are wonderful money-saving bargains. In these cases, the bargains will save you money if you do a little forward planning. But, before you decide to add the on-sale items to your cart, first ask yourself if you are going to have time to portion out and freeze some of the items, or if you are being persuaded by the price of the item. In the case that you will not take the time to portion out and freeze some, buying less would be a better decision.

An important tip for you to remember is that not every weight loss journey requires you to start from scratch. Whenever you have the opportunity, go through your pantry and cupboard to see what items you still have. Not only will you be able to rid yourself of some unnecessary or long-expired and unusable items, but you will be surprised how many of the items you already have can easily fulfill your macro needs. You may not need to stock up on as many food items as you once thought you'd need.

And finally, if you ever find yourself in the position of having leftovers, you can either repurpose the leftovers into a new meal or you could eat the leftovers as they are.

Meal Timing and Frequency

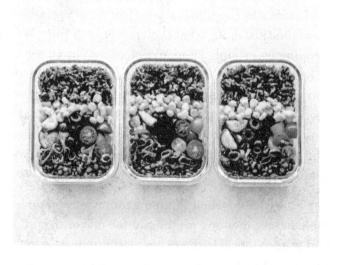

Aside from getting your macros just right and prepping your meals, you also need to consider when you eat. Let me give you an example: Do you know why it isn't recommended to eat a large meal or a carb-heavy meal right before bed? Well, eating any large meal, but especially one that is high in carbs, puts all this fuel into your body, but you don't use that fuel because you go to sleep. The fuel that isn't used or burned gets stored as fat. This is one of the more obvious examples, but consuming foods at specific times can make workouts and rest periods more beneficial for your weight loss journey.

When it comes to mealtimes, many people tend to vary greatly when they eat their meals. There are some diets or eating plans that people use, such as intermittent fasting which requires them to fast for a time, and then they have a window in which they can eat. In terms of counting macronutrients, the time in which you eat may also be a factor.

When it comes to eating dinner, we have already discussed why eating dinner too late is not ideal. If you eat dinner just before bed, there is not enough time between your meal and your rest for your body to burn off some of the energy that it has just consumed. Additionally, you may also find that your sleep is restless if you eat too late. The ideal time to eat dinner would be about two to three hours before you sleep. This doesn't mean that you should eat dinner at 8 p.m. if you go to bed at 10 p.m. Ideally, you should eat dinner by 5 p.m. or 6 p.m. to give your body a chance to use up that energy.

When it comes to lunch, this seems to be the meal that you can have more freedom with. Lunch doesn't seem to have as much of an impact on weight loss, and in most cases, it should be your largest meal of the day. The thing is, however, that society tends to make a bigger deal and a greater fuss of dinner, whereas breakfast and lunch usually provide your body with the fuel it needs to conquer the day, so to speak.

"Breakfast is the most important meal of the day." How many times have you heard that? Well, in terms of breakfast being important, I think there is a lot of flexibility surrounding when you consume your first meal of the day. As mentioned, there are people who do intermittent fasting, and they have their first meal at 11 a.m., and this has been shown to work wonders when it comes to weight loss for many people. Does this mean that eating breakfast at 7 a.m. is inherently incorrect? No, not at all. The important thing to remember is that there is a break between dinner the night before and the first meal of the day. This is where we see that meal timing is interlinked because having dinner earlier allows you to have a 12-hour break between one meal and the next. That way, your body burns calories, heals, repairs, and rests, and the next morning, whether it is at 7 a.m. or 11 a.m., you can have a nutrient-dense meal that gives you enough energy to tackle every task that comes your way.

To eat for weight loss, there are tips you can keep in mind (Williams, 2020):

1. Carbs give you energy, and protein heals and repairs muscles. Consume each meal, accordingly, depending on when you need your fuel and when you need repair work on your muscles after a workout.
2. Try to eat most of your meals or your larger meals during the earlier part of the day.
3. Keep dinner light and try to put 12 hours between dinner and breakfast.

You may have also heard that skipping meals or putting too much time between your meals may slow down your metabolism. However, studies have shown that meal frequency and how often you eat don't substantially impact your metabolic rate (Klein, 2015). As we have already established, weight loss can only come from a calorie deficit, and the best meal plan for you to follow is the one you can stick with. So, play around with your eating windows and find what works best for you.

Summary

- Meal prep, when done correctly, not only proves to be extremely beneficial for weight loss but also gives you more time in the day because it removes the mammoth task of preparing meals.
- It can also save you money.

- Meal prep, coupled with eating at the correct times, can really prove to enhance your weight loss strategy and yield results even quicker.

Now, while we know that meal prep is great, you may be wondering how you can create these ideal, balanced, and macronutrient-rich meals. Well, in the next chapter, we are going to break down how you can create balanced meals for your goals and your unique body type.

7

CREATING BALANCED MEALS THAT WORK FOR YOUR BODY TYPE

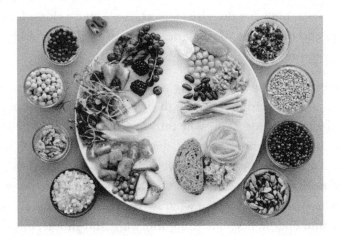

For the longest time, I have seen people go on highly restrictive crash diets that have them eating next to nothing and unable to enjoy food. They go for days barely eating anything, and when they do eventually run out of willpower and eat off plan, they usually overeat junk foods that make them feel defeated. The misconception or misunderstanding that you must starve yourself to lose weight needs to end, and embracing good foods that fill you up needs to replace that thinking.

I am sure that as you have read this book, the common theme and thread has made itself obvious. But if it has not, here it is: The reason counting macros is such an effective way of losing weight is that it helps you get the nutrients you need. When your goal is to lose weight, it is easy to get distracted by the deep seated need to consume less just so that you can lose weight or get to your target weight. However, it is extremely important to give our bodies nutritious meals that satisfy our nutritional needs. The last thing we want is to undo the hard work we put into weight loss because our body has gone into starvation mode. Additionally, the last thing anyone wants to do is develop an eating disorder because of an extremely restrictive diet.

This entire weight loss journey is all about balance—finding the balance and maintaining it. You may have heard the term "balanced meals" often, but what does this mean? As we take a closer look at the concept and the notion of a balanced meal, we will also find that each person requires their own type of balance.

Let's consider metabolism for a second. Metabolism has actually become a scary word that people throw around. It has become something that, if it is too slow, will cause us to gain weight or not lose weight. It has become so popular that, in fact, people search for ways to increase their metabolism. However, it is not as scary as the weight loss world has made it out to be. Our metabolism is the process that our bodies use to break down what we consume, in terms of food and drinks, into energy. It seems straightforward and simple, but truth be told, the last thing anyone wants to hear is that they have a slow metabolism.

However, based on the previous chapters where we looked at different body types, I think it has become plain to see that there are some body types that have inherently different metabolisms than others. The way each person metabolizes food is different, but also different foods are metabolized differently by different people. This makes the notion of metabolizing food that much more complex because when you think about it, everyone has a different metabolism.

Consider this for a second: Some people can eat dairy, and others get bloated and extremely uncomfortable if they eat dairy. Then there are others who can eat bread happily and others who could end up with severe stomach pain if they eat bread. Finally, there are people who can take pain pills, and they can go about their day as normal, but there are others who may take those exact same pills and are barely able to keep their eyes open. This happens because, genetically, each person is different, and these differences influence how our bodies break down and metabolize food.

That is why when you are combining and preparing meals to make sure you get all your macronutrients in, it is important to be aware of what foods agree with you and what foods don't agree with you. If someone is lactose intolerant, they may not include large portions of cheese, milk, or dairy as their fat macro each day. Instead, they may opt for nuts, avocado, and other fats that are more agreeable with their body.

How to Easily Combine Foods to Create Meals

There are just some food items that go together and others that just don't. Whether it is something like salted caramel, which just somehow works, or something like pineapple on pizza which just causes so much controversy, there are things that seem to go together and others that don't. While these are just examples of tastes and flavors, there are other things that seem to go together that pose health benefits when combined. For example, lemon and honey seem to boost endless health benefits, and there always seems to be a combination of foods, herbs, or spices that someone will tell you to take as a way of curing an ailment.

In the same way, there seem to be certain foods that, when combined, are thought to provide weight loss and weight management benefits.

Whether these food combinations aid in weight loss or they just enhance your digestive health, there are specific combinations that have gained traction and fame in the health and fitness circles.

Basically, food combining is the notion that when certain foods are consumed together, it may promote weight loss or enhance one's overall health. There are some food combining practices that seem quite complex and even hard to maintain. Then there are others that seem straightforward. Either way, we know that combining certain macros in specific amounts will prove to be beneficial (Ajmera, 2022).

What is important to note is that while there is no scientific evidence that different food combinations work for weight loss, eating certain combinations provide other indirect benefits that tend to help or push our bodies toward weight loss. For example, when you consider high blood sugar and the fact that many people who have diabetes can present as overweight or obese (not all the time, but in many instances), we can draw a link between blood sugar and weight. Scientifically, we can say that a combination of macronutrients stabilizes one's blood sugar and keeps it at an appropriate level for a long period of time (Ajmera, 2022).

Additionally, when you consume high-fat foods, you tend not to get hungry as quickly, meaning you snack less, and you find yourself better sustained by the whole balanced meal that you are eating. So, for that reason, while there is no direct scientific evidence that encourages you to mix lemon with honey and hot water for weight loss or that proves these combinations to be effective, choosing the correct ratios of macronutrients can sustain you and provide you with secondary benefits that promote weight loss. From reduced hunger to maintaining blood sugar levels, a balanced meal is a healthy meal.

Aside from these secondary benefits of weight loss that come with a balanced meal, you can also be sure that these meals provide you with everything your body yearns for. This means no deficiencies or risks of illness because you are not getting enough of a specific nutrient. Also, there are many restrictive diets that require you to eliminate certain foods, no matter how much you enjoy or like those foods. Now I don't know about you, but I am a sweets person. Any diet that required me to give up sweets entirely and forever was an enemy to me. This is because, at some point, I would take a "day off" from my diet. On my days off, I would overindulge in sweets because I felt deprived due to a really restrictive diet. There is an age-old saying that everything should be taken in moderation. Having a balanced diet allows this!

We know and have established and emphasized over the course of this book, that a well-balanced meal includes all three macronutrients in different ratios depending on your individual goals and body type. But if you are just starting this journey of counting your macros, you may find yourself wondering what balanced foods and combinations you can eat to start your journey. Well, something as simple as avocado and an egg on whole grain toast is a good start. You can have yogurt with fresh fruit and nuts or even salmon, rice, broccoli, and asparagus. If you are more of a sandwich or wrap person, you could find a balanced meal in a chicken, feta, and roast vegetable sandwich or wrap.

Since we have mentioned metabolism, you may be wondering if there are certain foods or food combinations that may speed up your metabolism. While these are not permanent fixes (because your metabolism isn't something that can be altered but can rather be fed certain things that are metabolized faster), you will find that a high protein diet generally promotes weight loss because of the way our bodies break down and use protein. If you are someone who has used a lot of diet plans and weight loss plans, you may have noticed that most of these plans make use of a high-protein diet.

If you are hoping to eat food specifically for weight loss, Felson (2022) suggests that combos are better than single foods because two are better than one. To lose weight, different nutrients in different foods can work together to keep you sustained even longer and can work together to burn calories better and faster. Combining leafy greens with avocado will fill you up more than just greens alone, adding cayenne pepper to chicken breasts may boost your metabolism and the protein will fill you up, yogurt with berries provides protein and fiber which are both known to help you feel less hungry, and adding beans to vegetable soup to make it more filling are all great ways of aiding in weight loss through food combos (Felson, 2022).

Meals for Each Body Type

Now that we know the intricacies of how each macronutrient works and interacts with each body type, you may be wondering what you can eat for your body type. After all, protein, fat, and carbs are just a broad description of over a thousand food and meal ideas. Where would you even begin? It can all seem extremely daunting and over-whelming, but what is this book, if not a helpful guide?

Foods for Endomorphs

We already know that endomorphs appear to hold more weight or fat, especially around their midsection. It is important to note that being an endomorph isn't what causes health issues, but rather the propensity to gain fat easily can usually lead to illnesses such as diabetes or insulin resistance. Because this body type carries more fat, the foods or macros that should be reduced are carbs so that fat loss can be promoted. Someone who has an endomorph body type probably has a slower metabolism because fat burns fewer calories than muscle. This means that by limiting carbs, you are not only even out your blood sugar levels but you also encourage your body to burn fat from its stores rather than from the energy sources that you are feeding your body through carbs.

Remember that mixing and matching meals and using different combinations of foods is a great way of keeping things fun and inter-esting despite being on a weight loss journey. Endomorph body types generally require their macros to come from 25% carbs, 35% proteins, and 40% fats.

Foods that endomorphs should be encouraged to eat are turkey meat, chicken, and salmon, under the meat and fish category. They can enjoy milk and yogurt as dairy products (and should probably stick to these rather than cheeses). In terms of fruits and vegetables, leafy greens are encouraged, and berries, pears, apples, onions, tomatoes, and zucchini can all be included in their meals (Migala, 2022b).

A variety of nuts and seeds can be enjoyed, such as nut butter, seed butter, sunflower and pumpkin seeds, and almonds and pistachios. In terms of grains, brown rice, quinoa, and oats are all great for endomorph consumption.

If you find yourself stuck or unable to come up with ideas of what to eat, why not consider yogurts and berries, apples covered in nut butter, or oats with milk for breakfast? As a lunch option, you could try turkey meat with zucchini fries or a chicken salad that is packed with leafy greens. When you realize just how varied your options are, it can easily feel like you're not even on a diet despite appearing as though the odds are stacked up against you by having an endomorph body type. Do you know what the best part is? You will still lose weight and enjoy feeling healthier and better!

As mentioned earlier, a simple way to start your meal plan would be to begin with 2-6 ounces of protein or the equivalent of 14-42 grams of protein (breakfast could have a small amount of protein, lunch could have a large amount, and dinner could have a moderate amount using these guidelines), 4-6 ounces of fruit (or about 100 calories of something starchy if you are really having a craving), 4-6 ounces of vegetables (this can be omitted for breakfast), and maybe some added fat, and then adjust up or down to fit your macronutrient ratios and caloric needs.

Although I cannot create a meal plan for you because counting macros is very individualized, I will give you some ideas to help get you thinking.

Following are examples of meals that are close to the 25% carbs, 35% protein, and 40% fat recommended for the endomorph body type and are based on a 1,200-calorie intake.

All are estimates, based on common brands listed in the My Fitness Pal application. Please carefully check your own foods to get accurate information for your daily food intake.

Example 1

Breakfast: small apple, mushrooms and spinach omelet made with 1 egg and 3 Tbsp. egg whites and 1 oz. cheddar cheese

Lunch: 4 oz. strawberries, 5 oz. salmon, 4 oz. steamed asparagus with 2 Tbsp. butter

Dinner: 4 oz. cantaloupe, 2 oz. ground turkey with 2 oz. ground sirloin, 4 oz. zucchini noodles, ½ cup marinara sauce, 1 Tbsp. parmesan cheese, 1 Hawaiian sweet roll

Example 2

Breakfast: 1 cup of 2% cottage cheese, 4 oz. blueberries

Lunch: 5 oz. chicken breast, ¾ cups stir fry vegetables, 1 Tbsp. olive oil, 1/3 cup brown rice

Dinner: 5 oz. sirloin steak, 1 cup mixed greens salad, ½ a medium avocado, low-fat French dressing, 4 oz. orange

Example 3

Breakfast: 2 egg frittata with tomatoes, onions, and spinach, 3 Tbsp. guacamole, 4 oz. Cherries

Lunch: 5 oz. grilled chicken breast, 4 oz. spring mix lettuce, 5 cherry tomatoes, 2 oz. mozzarella cheese, 2 Tbsp. tzatziki sauce, 4 oz. Mandarin oranges

Dinner: pecan encrusted cod cooked in 1 Tbsp. olive oil with ¼ cup pecans and egg white, 4 oz. broccoli, 4 oz. raspberries

Example 4 (planning for a party)

Breakfast: protein shake, 4 oz. strawberries

Lunch: 5 oz. pork loin chops, 4 oz. applesauce, 4 oz. green beans, 2 Tbsp. Butter

Dinner: about 2 oz. gouda cheese, about 4 oz. celery dipped in about 2 oz. Guacamole, ½ medium sized piece of chocolate cake

Remember to drink plenty of water throughout the day and adjust the portion sizes or consult a registered dietitian if you have specific dietary needs or health concerns.

Foods for Ectomorphs

There are two schools of thought when it comes to ectomorphs who want to lose weight. Some say they should use the macronutrient ratios for endomorphs, while others say they should use the macronutrient ratios for ectomorphs because their body will still react the way an ectomorph body typically reacts. For me personally, I had to use the macronutrient ratios for an ectomorph before I started seeing results. So, if your body resembled an ectomorph before you put on weight, using ectomorph ratios may be the best way to get started.

As mentioned earlier in the book, the ideal ratio of macro consumption for an ectomorph is for around 55% of their macros to come from carbs, 25% to come from protein, and 20% to come from fats.

For an ectomorph, carbohydrates are their friends. Consuming foods such as brown rice, brown pasta, and potatoes are ways of getting the good carbs in, and that allows the body to create energy in a healthy way. Additionally, if an ectomorph is trying to build muscle, they need to consume enough protein, which contributes to muscle development. The best types of protein that an ectomorph can consume are lean steak, eggs, protein shakes, fish, turkey, and chicken (Johnson, 2020).

When it comes to fats, this is where ectomorphs need to be slightly more careful because although they need fat for muscle growth, their bodies don't always show when they are consuming too much fat. So, while there may be a buildup of fat in their arteries and deep in their subcutaneous tissue, it may not be obvious for a long time. Sticking to the healthy fats such as omega 3, 6, and 9, flaxseed oil, avocado, and fish are great fats for ectomorphs to consume.

As mentioned earlier, a simple way to start your meal plan would be to begin with 2-6 ounces of protein or the equivalent of 14-42 grams of protein (breakfast could have a small amount of protein, lunch could have a large amount, and dinner could have a moderate amount using these guidelines), 4-6 ounces of fruit (or about 100 calories of something starchy), 4-6 ounces of vegetables (this can be omitted for breakfast), and maybe some added fat, and then adjust up or down to fit your macronutrient ratios and caloric needs.

Although I cannot create a meal plan for you because counting macros is very individualized, I will give you some ideas to help get you thinking.

Following are examples of meals that are close to the 55% carbs, 25% protein, and 20% fat recommended for the ectomorph body type and are based on a 1,200-calorie intake.

All are estimates, based on common brands listed in the My Fitness Pal application. Please carefully check your own foods to get accurate information for your daily food intake.

Example 1

Breakfast: 4 oz. egg white omelet with 2 oz. mushrooms and 2 oz. onions, 2 Tbsp. salsa, ½ English muffin, 4 oz. apple

Lunch: 4 oz. pork loin, 4 oz. sauerkraut, 4 oz. broccoli, 4 oz. cherries, small whole wheat roll

Dinner: 4 oz. ground beef, 4 oz. marinara sauce, 4 oz. spaghetti noodles, 4 oz. green beans, 4 oz. mandarin oranges, 1 small whole wheat roll.

Example 2

Breakfast: 4 oz. of 2% cottage cheese, 5 oz. blueberries, 1 slice whole what toast, 1 Tbsp. butter

Lunch: 3 oz. turkey burger patty, 1 whole wheat bun, 2 oz. tomatoes, 2 oz. red onion, lettuce, mustard, 3 oz. baby carrots, 1 medium pear

Dinner: 3 oz. sirloin steak, 4 oz. asparagus, small baked potato, 5 oz. watermelon, 1 cup mixed greens salad, 1 Tbsp. ranch dressing, 1 Tbsp. butter

Example 3

Breakfast: 1 small banana, 1 cup oatmeal with a splash of skim milk

Lunch: 2 cups mixed greens salad, 4 oz. tomatoes, 4 oz. cucumber, 3 oz. chicken breast, 2 Tbsp. lite balsamic vinaigrette, 1 medium apple

Dinner: 4 oz. salmon, 4 oz. broccoli, 4 oz. quinoa, 4 oz. strawberries

Example 4 (planning for a party)

Breakfast: 1 cup of oatmeal with a splash of skim milk, 4 oz. strawberries

Lunch: 4 oz. pork loin chops, 5 oz. applesauce, 4 oz. green beans with balsamic vinegar, small whole wheat roll

Dinner (party foods): about 20 pretzels dipped in 2 Tbsp hummus, about 20 grapes, 3 slices of turkey meat on two Hawaiian rolls with mustard

Remember to drink plenty of water throughout the day and adjust the portion sizes or consult a registered dietitian if you have specific dietary needs or health concerns.

Foods For Mesomorphs

Mesomorphs are people who can typically change the way their body looks fairly quickly when they adjust what they eat. When a mesomorph puts on excess weight, it is usually because they have been eating more carbs or fat than their body can properly process. If this is the case, the mesomorph should adjust their food intake to be more balanced. For the most part, if a mesomorph is already pretty healthy and they are hoping to maintain their body, they can stick to a relatively balanced diet whereby each of their macros are consumed in almost equal quantities. This means that about 40% of their diet can come from carbs, 30% from fats, and 30% from proteins. If they want to gain more muscle, they can increase their protein, and if they are hoping to gain weight, they can increase their carbs. They can also use the general rule of thumb by making sure each meal has about 4 to 6 ounces of protein, fruits, and vegetables in their diet, and adjusting according to their goals as it changes.

In terms of meat and fish that mesomorphs should eat, nothing is really off limits, provided that they eat everything in moderation. Turkey, steak, chicken, eggs, fish, and even protein shakes are great sources of protein. When it comes to dairy, they can enjoy their share of yogurts and cheeses. They also get to enjoy a wide variety of fruits, vegetables, nuts, seeds, and grains (Migala, 2022a).

As mentioned earlier, a simple way to start your meal plan would be to begin with 2-6 ounces of protein or the equivalent of 14-42 grams of protein (breakfast could have a small amount of protein, lunch could have a large amount, and dinner could have a moderate amount using these guidelines), 4-6 ounces of fruit (or about 100 calories of something starchy), 4-6 ounces of vegetables (this can be omitted for breakfast), and maybe some added fat, and then adjust up or down to fit your macronutrient ratios and caloric needs.

Although I cannot create a meal plan for you because counting macros is very individualized, I will give you some ideas to help get you thinking.

Following are examples of meals that are close to the 40% carbs, 30% protein, and 30% fat recommended for the ectomorph body type and are based on a 1,200-calorie intake.

All are estimates, based on common brands listed in the My Fitness Pal application. Please carefully check your own foods to get accurate information for your daily food intake.

Example 1

Breakfast: 4 oz. scrambled egg whites cooked with non-stick spray, 1 slice of whole-grain toast, 4 oz. of mixed berries, 2 Tbsp. butter

Lunch: 4 oz. Grilled chicken breast, 1 cup of mixed greens, 4 oz. of cherry tomatoes, 4 oz. of cucumber, 2 tablespoons of ranch dressing, medium apple

Dinner: 4 oz. baked salmon, 1/2 cup of quinoa, 4 oz. of steamed broccoli, 1/2 cup of Greek yogurt sweetened with stevia or monk fruit, 4 oz. of blueberries

Example 2

Breakfast: 1 cup of oatmeal with a splash of skim milk, 4 oz. strawberries, 4 slices of turkey bacon

Lunch: 5 oz. of turkey breast slices wrapped in lettuce leaves, 3 oz baby carrots, mustard, small orange

Dinner: 5 oz. grilled sirloin steak, 1/2 cup of brown rice, 4 oz. of roasted Brussels sprouts, 4 oz. of cucumber slices, 2 tablespoons of tzatziki sauce, 4 oz. applesauce

Example 3

Breakfast: 2 egg omelet with 2 oz. spinach and 1 oz. mushrooms, topped with 1 oz. salsa and cooked with non-stick spray, 1 slice of whole-grain toast, 1 small pear, 1 Tbsp. cashew butter

Lunch: Chicken and chickpea salad: 3 oz. grilled chicken breast, 4 oz. of canned chickpeas, 1 oz. diced celery, 1 oz. diced red onion, 1 cup lettuce, 2 Tbsp. ranch dressing, 4 oz. of cherry tomatoes

Dinner: 5 oz. grilled shrimp, small baked potato, 1 cup of steamed asparagus, 4oz. of 2% cottage cheese, 4 oz. of pineapple chunks

Example 4 (planning for a party)

Breakfast: 1 cup Greek yogurt sweetened with stevia or monk fruit, 1/4 cup of granola, 4 oz. of mixed berries

Lunch: 5 oz. grilled chicken breast, 1 cup of mixed greens, 4 oz. of cherry tomatoes, 4 oz. of cucumber, 2 tablespoons of balsamic vinaigrette, 3 oz. orange wedges

Dinner (party foods): Hamburger on a half a bun with mustard and veggies (no cheese), ½ cup of chocolate ice cream

Remember to drink plenty of water throughout the day and adjust the portion sizes or consult a registered dietitian if you have specific dietary needs or health concerns.

Now that you have the wealth of information, it is time for you to start playing around with meal ideas. Something that you can do is get yourself a planner, whether it is a weekly or monthly planner, and you can start playing with meal combinations and meal ideas. Start with one week, where you create meal ideas according to your required macros for each day. Mix and match combinations, and through the help of your macro tracking app, you can see what proteins can be swapped out in each meal, and you can see what carbs and fats can be alternated to create balanced, healthy, and different meals each time.

Preparing to endeavor on a weight loss journey is never easy. The reality is that motivation ebbs and flows. There are going to be times when you won't want to do anything. I have come to learn that there are two types of people: those who lose weight or see results, and these results encourage them to continue, and those who lose weight or see results and see an excuse to reward themselves with junk which ultimately sets them back. To be honest, I've been both of those people at different points in my life.

Some days will be easy, and some days will be hard. Some days, you won't want to stick to your meal plans, and on those days, you will need an extra push. In the next chapter, we are going to look at how you can stay motivated or at least find motivation on the harder days. We are also going to look at the obstacles you may face and how you can overcome those obstacles each day.

8

STAYING MOTIVATED AND OVERCOMING OBSTACLES

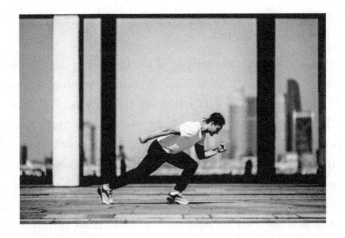

Many people think that all you need to lose weight is a bit of willpower and motivation. To those people, I say you need far more than just a bit. In fact, staying healthy is hard to do. I can guarantee you that there are always going to be reasons why you shouldn't, why you can't, or why you just don't feel like it. But once you find a greater purpose behind why you are trying to lose weight and stay healthy, you may find motivation slightly easier to come by.

A lot of people that I know who have ventured on a weight loss journey have found permanent reasons to motivate them. You see, losing weight for a wedding or for an event is temporary. After the event passes, what reason do you have to maintain a healthy lifestyle? But when people are motivated by things like spending time with their kids or when they are motivated by living long enough to see their grandkids, they have a life-long motivation.

To achieve your weight loss goals, you need motivation. If you had no motivation, you would have no need to lose weight. But how do you maintain the motivation long-term without it deteriorating over time? How do you make sure that you stick to your healthy lifestyle, whether you are on vacation, at a party, or at special dinners? I mean, you know how easy it is to agree to a second piece of cake at a birthday party and how easy it is to take two donuts instead of one. We are going to take a deeper look at the tactics you should employ to avoid feeling demotivated.

There is an old saying that tells us if we love what we do, we never work a day in our lives. Well, this is something that is known as intrinsic motivation, and it is when we find joy in the actual task rather than hoping for the task to yield some form of result (Oudeyer & Kaplan, 2007). It is the notion that you enjoy doing something so much that the fact that it yields positive benefits is just a bonus and not the actual motivating reason behind why you are doing that task. For example, there are people who run for the pure joy of it. They run because of how clear their minds are when they're running, how relaxed they feel, and how happy they are with the wind in their hair. In many cases, you will find that these people who run are rarely ever motivated to run by the number of the scale, and because this task is so enjoyable for them, they don't even need to go on the scale because the very thing that is bringing them joy is keeping them healthy. Ideally, this is where you want to be in terms of counting your macros and carrying out your meal prep. Being organized and having balanced meals ready quickly needs to become so enjoyable that you actually find a sense of satisfaction in the prep of your meals and that weight loss is just a natural benefit.

I get it, though, not everyone finds enjoyment in such things, but this doesn't mean that there isn't some other part of your weight loss journey (aside from actually losing weight) in which you could find intrinsic motivation.

The Importance of Staying Motivated for Long-Term Success

So how do you become intrinsically motivated, especially when you're not losing weight for an event or a situation? Intrinsic motivation actually comes down to mindfulness and an active awareness of doing something for the now. So, in the moment if you feel deprived while you eat the well-balanced meal that you've prepared as opposed to the burger and fries that your friends are having for lunch, remind yourself that this is about now. It isn't about being skinny next week or next month, but it is about being healthy right now, in this moment. When you set your sights on a day-by-day approach, you may find it easier to stay motivated as opposed to placing the weight of a mammoth long-term goal on your shoulders.

But to make this even easier to do, there are some steps that you can follow (Nguyen, 2022):

- We have already discussed the notion of setting SMART goals. If you are going to find an intrinsic motivation that comes from the process of losing weight, it is important to be realistic about your goals. Wanting to lose 15 pounds for your wedding that's a month away is not realistic. Setting such a goal is just going to make you feel miserable when you don't reach that goal, or you see yourself falling short just a week into your weight loss journey.
- We know that in a macro-tracking lifestyle, you are doing just that—tracking everything. Record what you eat, when you eat, how you exercise, when you exercise, and everything

in between. This not only makes you accountable because you are forced to record what you have eaten, whether it was healthy or not, but you also get to see what you enjoy eating and what exercises you enjoy doing, and you can better stick to your healthy lifestyle by focusing on the things you actually enjoy.

- When you find yourself feeling slightly demotivated, motivate yourself. Give yourself a pep talk. While weight loss is always great in a community or a team, the reality is that you are the only person who is always going to be with you. Having people around you can motivate you, but it only works when you're with those people. If you are motivated by yourself and the positive self-talk you can give yourself; then you can remain motivated even when you are alone.

- The combination of a schedule or checklist, together with a weight-loss journal, can be incredibly powerful. On one side, you can schedule everything that you need to do as part of your weight loss journey, and in your journal, you can record whether or not you have completed these tasks and how you felt when you did so. You also get to track your progress when you record everything, and before you know it, you will look back and see how far you have come, and you will be proud of yourself.

- As previously mentioned, it is always great to do the things you enjoy. If you prefer high-impact training and heavy lifting, go for CrossFit workouts. If you like high-speed workouts and working up a sweat, then opt for running and all the joys that come with a cardio workout. And if you prefer a calmer and lower-impact workout, you could consider exercises like yoga and Pilates. Ultimately, you need to do what you enjoy, and you need to align that with your goals.

- While you do need to find motivation within yourself, never underestimate the role of a support team and have like-minded people around you.

Overcoming Common Obstacles When Counting Macros

There are so many things that can derail us from a diet or an eating plan. But you know what's even harder than facing the weekend when you're on a diet? Doing things that are out of your routine when you're pursuing a lifestyle change. The things that are supposed to be enjoyable, like a birthday dinner at a restaurant with your family, become something that terrifies you because you don't know how you are going to track your macros while you're out.

The reality is that some things are out of your scope of knowledge. If you're invited to a birthday party, and Susan makes her famous chocolate fudge cake, you may have an idea of what ingredients are in there, but if she tells you it's her super special secret recipe, you may not know if it is condensed milk, chocolate chips, or even mayonnaise. And in some cases, you have to allow the unknown to happen and relinquish control of the things you can't control. But that doesn't mean you can't take a guess and add in what you already know.

If you are heading out to a restaurant for dinner, one of the best things you can do is check the menu beforehand. You can look at the size of their servings if you are hoping to have a steak or something similar, you can look at the sides that come with each dish, and you and your app can estimate how many macros you are expected to consume. Not only does this make tracking your macros much easier, but it also makes it easier for you to plan your macros ahead of time. If you know that you're heading out for brunch, you could adjust what you're going to have for dinner to accommodate your brunch plans.

There are a few places that prove easier for tracking macros than others. As a rule of thumb, it is always safe to assume that any place that prepares your meal from scratch is probably easier for tracking your macros than a place that has a drive-through. This means that fast foods are not great for macro tracking, and they also won't have much quality to the calories you are consuming. It is easier for you to track the macros in a 200g rack of ribs with salt and pepper and a side of a baked potato. You also need to consider things such as dips, sauces, bastings, and other things that usually slip our minds when we're eating.

While there are unavoidable situations, it is always best to limit how often you head out to eat. When you prepare meals at home, you know exactly what is going into your meal. There are also some logical calls that you can make when you're heading out to a social gathering. At a birthday party, you won't likely find baby carrots and hummus as a dip or a wide array of steak and lean meat cuts. Instead, you will find foods that are high in carb and fat macros. You can compensate for this by eating the macros at home that you aren't likely to find at the party. If you are worried about your macros when you are heading out on vacation, the easiest thing you can do is plan ahead. You're going to want to make sure that you have meals and snacks planned and prepared, so that you can limit your convenience store stops.

Keeping Yourself Accountable

As previously mentioned, accountability comes from many different sources. It can come from yourself, or it can come from others. It is always great to have someone to whom you can be accountable but knowing that you have yourself to answer to makes it that much easier to stick to your plan and reach your goals.

Accountability can be hard. It is something that most people struggle with. But luckily, there are hacks and tricks that you can use to maintain your accountability.

Let's be honest, there are different forms of accountability that exist. Let us consider our professional lives. If you work, you have a boss or a manager that keeps you accountable by checking your work and making sure that everything you do is up to standard. If you are your own boss or you run an organization, you are accountable to yourself, but you are also accountable to the people you employ or the people that make use of your services. This means that if you don't work, you and your employees may not see an income.

If you have a family or you have kids, you may find that you are accountable to them to make sure that there is always food, that they are always well taken care of, that they are clothed, and that they have a decent place to live. Somehow, in the list of things to be accountable for, our own health tends to be last on the list. It is also the one thing that actually requires some form of accountability and even a sense of responsibility.

But since weight loss and our health is one of the hardest places to find and maintain accountability, it is here where I am going to give you a few tips on finding and maintaining your accountability.

Accountability is usually strongly found in the milestones that we reach on our way to our goals. Our progress is what keeps us motivated to keep pushing. It starts with something as simple as recording what you are eating and what you are doing. Tomorrow when you feel like eating a cookie instead of an apple, you can look back on the previous day and be reminded of who you were yesterday. I guarantee you that nothing makes you want to be a better you than trying to be better than a past version of yourself.

Next, employing a team is a sure way of getting you to where you want to be. I am not just talking about gym partners and accountability partners, but I am talking about telling your family members what you are doing and what you are hoping to achieve, because they will typically call you out if they see you falling off the wagon even slightly. It also means adding a professional or an expert to your team or your support group. Having a doctor or a nutritionist whom you can engage often will not only keep you accountable because you have someone waiting and expecting results, but it will also help you in knowing and understanding when you need to make changes to what you are doing.

You're also going to want to weigh and measure yourself regularly. Some people do so every day, but this could lead to you not seeing results in such a short time and maybe feeling worse off. If you weigh and measure yourself once a week, you are more likely to have something great to show for your hard work.

One thing that has kept me motivated and that I have seen a lot of people on social media use as a means of accountability is a "skinny outfit." I had a pair of jeans that I really liked but that I had long outgrown. My goal became to fit into those jeans again. It started with getting them up my thighs. Then I worked harder to get them up to my waist. Then I carried on until I could zip them halfway up. Finally, I was able to button them, and I had reached a big goal. Having a "skinny outfit" gives you a clothing item to be accountable to. Just be sure to take pictures of your progress so that you can be reminded of how far you've come.

And finally, you can create a rewards system or point program for yourself. If you reach a certain milestone, you can get yourself something you really like. If you reach a specific weight by a certain time, then you can take yourself shopping or reward yourself with something you really enjoy. There are many people who choose to reward themselves with a cheat meal. And while that is perfectly fine, it is something that I have actively avoided because I found that all too often, a cheat meal would turn into a cheat weekend, and that could turn into a cheat week, and instead of maintaining accountability, it left me off the wagon and worse off than where I was. For most people, rewarding themselves with a non-food item is best. I had a friend who absolutely loved candles. She had a certain type of candle that she enjoyed purchasing for herself, and every time she reached a milestone, she would spoil herself with a candle. Other non-food rewards could be streaming a movie, grabbing a lottery ticket, buying a new book, or getting fresh flowers for the house. The reward doesn't have to be big, just enjoyable. Find something that you like and that you enjoy, and spoil yourself every time you achieve something you never thought you could.

Celebrating Your Successes and Staying Positive

There are definitely days when your new lifestyle can seem more like a chore than a pleasure. It is on these days when it can seem nearly impossible to stay positive. I can assure you that even the greatest athletes and nutrition coaches have been in this exact same position. This is normal and often comes with the fatigue of trying to accomplish too much at once.

A lot of the time, as soon as we reach one goal, we already begin setting the next. We create momentum and feel that while we are winning, we should set the next goal so that we can win at that too. But sometimes, what we need to do is take a second to be proud of ourselves and enjoy what we have already achieved. In a health and weight loss journey, this can look like reaching your goal or target weight and then immediately hopping onto a new goal of building muscle and toning up. Instead of congratulating yourself for the hard work and effort you have put in to come this far, you immediately move on to the next thing.

But celebrating your success is so important. This is because when you celebrate your wins, you create feelings of gratitude, compassion, and pride. These feelings are stronger than willpower and even the guilt that often pushes us to do certain things. When you have these positive emotions as the wind in your sails, you are more likely to set yourself up for future success. You enter into a mindset of knowing that you can do something because you have already achieved your goals in the past. That is why taking a short break and celebrating your success is important.

Above we have looked at the notion of a point system or reward system that you can set up for yourself to celebrate your goals, but it is important to draw a line between celebrating and rewarding yourself. When you reward yourself, you may give your mind the impression that you no longer have anything to work toward because you have achieved the goal and you have reached the end of the process. This is usually what causes people to go back to their ways of old and undo all of the progress they have made. However, when you cele-brate yourself, you are mindful of the process that it takes to reach the goal, rather than the goal itself. Because you are mindful of the work and effort that you have put into achieving a goal, it makes it easier to appreciate that hard work and to do whatever you can to maintain it (Clarke, 2021). So, making rewards short and simple, but taking a little extra time to celebrate in a mindful way tends to be most effective.

It is also important to draw the line between celebrating in a healthy way and celebrating in a self-destructive way. Celebrating in a healthy way can mean including others in your success (because success is contagious), reflecting on how far you've come instead of just focusing on where you currently are, and really taking the time to show yourself appreciation. It is a human norm to celebrate others, and it is a beautiful thing to do. But we often forget to do it for ourselves too. So next time you reach a goal or milestone, or even if you have simply successfully counted your macros for three days in a row or created a detailed meal plan for the week, take a moment to appreciate yourself and your hard work.

A big part of celebrating success is positive thinking. The entire notion of celebrating one's success is about thinking about oneself in a positive manner. So, through the process of embracing positive thinking, take the time to notice how you feel. Do you feel like you have more energy? What is a notable change between before your weight loss journey and now? Are you sleeping better?

Then you need to take note of your clothes. Do you feel any different? If so, what is it that feels different? Do you see any other physical differences? Maybe your chin seems narrower, or your cheeks seem smaller. Does your hair look any different? Have your nails stopped breaking? These are the changes that are easily overlooked, but when we're reminded of them, we realize just how far we have come.

Now you may be asking why such an emphasis has been placed on staying motivated through a meal plan, weight loss journey, or tracking macros, and the answer is simple: Tracking macros can be a hard adjustment at first. It can be difficult to log every meal, snack, and drink that you consume. But what is worth it, is the way you feel, the way you move differently, and the way you can keep up with your kids and play on the playground with them. It is the change in life that the benefits bring. The reason why I am trying so hard to encourage you to stick to counting your macros is that I have seen the benefits it has posed for me, and others like me.

I also know how frustrating it can be to put in all the work and all the effort only to find that you have made minimal progress in the few weeks that you have been counting your macros. The reality is that because each person is so different, you may not stroll straight into weight loss by counting your macros. Instead, you may need to adjust your ratios slightly or change your workouts before you start to see results. But what I am telling you is that sticking with it is one of the most worthwhile things you will ever do because ten days, ten months, and ten years from now, you will be thanking yourself!

Facing challenges along any road is inevitable. In the next and final chapter of this book, we are going to look at some of the challenges you may encounter on this weight loss journey; we are going to look at how you can figure out what the issue is and how to overcome the issue. And finally, we will address a few of the frequently asked questions that come with macro tracking.

9

TROUBLESHOOTING AND FAQS

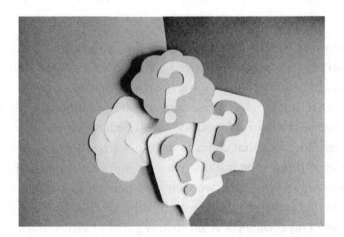

W eight loss is a tricky one. Many people pursue their dream body for their whole lives, while others seem to just have it served to them on a platter. In many cases, with the fast pace of life that we are currently living in, many people choose speed or convenience over health. This is because healthy choices are often the harder choices. Even those who seem to have willpower as strong as lead seem to face challenges on their weight loss journey.

In this chapter, let's take a look at some of the challenges and issues that you are bound to face on your weight loss journey, whether you are using the macro tracking method or any other weight loss method, there will be challenges such as weight loss plateaus. With a little knowledge, you can overcome these challenges.

I can almost guarantee you that at any given point, in any room full of people, there are at least a handful of them who are unhappy with or who are trying to do something about their weight. In most cases, there are more people who want to lose weight than there are people who are happy with their weight or who want to gain weight. I think the reason weight loss has become such a normal part of everyday conversation is because it is, in fact, so hard to do. If we could lose weight at will, it would be a nonissue. Because it is neither easy nor straightforward, we tend to face a lot of challenges on the way, but we can take comfort in knowing that these challenges can be overcome.

We know that you need to have goals before you embark on a weight loss journey. We have emphasized setting SMART goals and being realistic about what you're hoping to achieve and when you're hoping to achieve it. But in a lot of cases, we set our ambitions too high, and this becomes the reason for our downfall and our demise. Because of the weight loss fads that claim to be "quick fixes" for weight loss, we expect everything to be instant. After all, we live in a world of instant gratification, so why can't we drop the pounds instantly too? The reality is that most people give up healthy *lifestyles* because they set goals based on *crash diets*. A lifestyle is going to give you a slow and gradual change that can last a lifetime, but a crash diet is for now. When you embark on your macro-tracking journey, you need to know that you probably aren't going to see results immediately. However, by giving your body the proper nutrition, you should start feeling better fairly quickly. Once we accept and learn to trust the process, it will remove the option of giving up.

We can also add to the list of why people fail at weight loss: the fact that people fail to appreciate their bodies, tend to eat with their emotions, and that sometimes weight loss becomes their only goal to such an extent that they ignore basic nutrition and health. But despite these daunting challenges, there are ways of overcoming them and claiming back your health.

Overcoming a Weight Loss Plateau

No matter what means of weight loss you are pursuing, chances are that at some point, you are going to reach a weight loss plateau. Now, one of two things can happen: adjustments can be made for you to continue your success, or you can feel like you have failed, and you can give up. But before you make the decision, it is important that you are educated on what a weight loss plateau is.

A weight loss plateau is something everyone will face at some point in their life. It is the point when, despite maintaining a healthy lifestyle and strictly sticking to the plan that has been working successfully until now, you find yourself seemingly stuck, unable to move past your current weight, and you are not at your target or goal weight as yet.

In simple terms, your body reaches a plateau when it becomes used to diet or the exercise program that you are currently on. We know that there are many systems in the body that work together for weight loss to happen. Your muscles work to help you burn calories; you consume fewer calories so that your body uses its fat stores for energy and so much more. But when you have the initial drop in weight, it is important to remember that you are not only losing fat but muscle mass too. The less muscle mass you have, the less opportunity you have to burn fat (Mayo Clinic, 2018). The only way for you to move past the plateau is to change what you are already doing. This means that you need to change your workout by either increasing reps, moving from beginner to intermediate, or increasing the frequency of your workouts, or you can cut your calories further. If you choose to stick with what you are already doing, you will find that you maintain weight consistently (Mayo Clinic, 2018).

Additional ways of getting over the plateau are to increase your protein and cut down some carbs (or simply put, adjust your macros), make a note of any changes in your life that may be causing stress (this can impact weight loss and weight gain), try to include a means of intermittent fasting into your macro tracking, this would mean giving yourself a specific window of time in which to eat so that your body has enough time to enter ketosis which is the process where your body burns fat stores instead of glucose for energy (Cleveland Clinic, 2022), reduce your alcohol intake, and try to add more activity into your day (Spritzler, 2017).

On the note of adding more activity to your day, you may be concerned about adding more time to your exercise routine. After all, no one wants to spend hours at the gym. But you can introduce activity into your life in an unnoticeable way. Simple things like parking your car a bit further from the store entrance, taking the stairs instead of the elevator, and walking places instead of driving are great ways of introducing more activity into your life.

When you reach a plateau, it is also the place where it is easiest to fall off the wagon. The important thing is to identify that you are at a plateau and not use this as an excuse to give up on your healthy eating habits. This is most certainly not the time to give yourself an excuse to go back to old habits.

Keeping Up the Energy

The start of every eating plan or diet promises increased energy and a whole new outlook on life. But sometimes, we face a dip in that energy once we have been on a weight loss plan for a while. Perhaps it is not an energy dip per se, but we miss the energy boost we experienced at the start of the diet.

There are ways to limit the energy crash or the fatigue that you may face when you become accustomed to an eating plan. First, you can try to keep your meals small and rapid. This means that your body will be supplied with energy almost consistently, and it won't get fatigued in an attempt to preserve energy. Next, remember that even if you are trying to lose weight, you can utilize caffeine as a way of overcoming any slump you may face. Not only will you get an energy boost, but you may also have fewer calories to add to your daily log as caffeine is an appetite suppressant.

Throughout this book, we have looked at what foods add to the macros you need, but what we may have overlooked is foods that not only fall into these macros but that also provide you with a phenomenal source of energy. We all have days where we feel slightly lower than other days. This could be because of expected hormonal changes, changes in our routines, or even stress that caused us a restless night's sleep. But there are ways that you can use your plate to give you a boost.

The first thing you want to do is stay away from processed foods. This means that the last thing you should be eating is a fast-food burger and fries because the nutritional value is low. This will add to the fatigue rather than remedying it.

Next, as much as this may cause you to roll your eyes and say, "I know," having fresh fruits and vegetables will be sure to add to your energy and will make you feel happier and lighter. Lean proteins, whole grains, seeds and nuts, bananas, and oats are all great energy sources that can easily fit into and accommodate your macro-tracking lifestyle.

Then there is the master of energy—water. You see, the signs of dehydration aren't as glaringly obvious as we'd like them to be, and usually, we don't even realize we're dehydrated until we chug a glass of water and realize how refreshed and energized we are. One surefire way of avoiding dehydration is to drink water consistently throughout the day. This way, you don't even give your body a chance to dehydrate.

Many people think that they can boost their energy with an energy drink. But this should be avoided at all costs. If you are drinking a high-energy drink and you aren't burning that energy off, you may find yourself storing that energy as fat, and ultimately, you will be undoing all of your weight loss efforts. Because you are getting your calories from the energy drink instead of nutritious foods, you will still feel hungry, which could cause you to overeat. So, despite eating a healthy meal, you may gain weight. In the pursuit of health and weight loss, energy drinks should be avoided at all costs.

While this book has focused on macronutrients, it is pertinent that we do not forget that everything we need may not come from our food. Micronutrients, vitamins, and minerals are all part of a balanced diet, and just because we are consuming enough macros doesn't mean we should neglect the little things that we need. This is why I always recommend that people take a multivitamin to make up for the small things that we may not be getting from our foods, and we may not even be thinking about. After all, we want to be healthy during our weight loss journey, and we don't want to experience or develop any deficiencies.

Macro Tracking FAQs

1. Is macro tracking effective for vegetarians? Remember that protein doesn't just come from meat. There are endless numbers of plant-based proteins that you can use while still maintaining your vegetarian and vegan stance. It is important, however, to be aware of your micronutrients and make sure that you are getting vitamins like B12.
2. What if you don't hit your macros in a day? Remember that you are human, and life happens. If you are not as hungry as you usually are, which can happen, and you find that you don't hit your macros in the day, that is fine. As long as you are not changing your numbers based on one day's targets, it is fine to fall slightly short of your macros if need be.

3. Can you use a protein supplement? Basically, as long as you are counting it and tracking the macros you consume from the protein supplement, you can definitely have a protein shake.

4. What should you look for on a food label? The main items that you are going to be looking at on the seemingly endless list on the back of every food item are the calories, protein, carbs, and fat on the label. These are listed in grams and can be subtracted from the number you are allowed to consume in a day.

5. What if you are eating fresh foods that don't have a label? From the internet to your new closest friend—your macro tracking app, all the nutritional information for fresh foods will be listed. All you need to do is know the weight of the food you're eating. This is because natural and unprocessed foods are pretty consistent. Every ounce of a banana is going to have the exact same nutritional information no matter where you are.

Summary

Most days, it may seem like a breeze to be counting your macros, and other days, it may seem like you're barely keeping your head above water, but now that you have the tools needed to overcome the plateau, to maintain your energy, and to keep yourself healthy, you can begin this journey of health.

AFTERWORD

Not only have you learned what macronutrients are, but you have also learned how to use them to your benefit and as a means of weight loss. We have looked at the why and the how of counting macros from a scientific perspective, we have seen how you can use and manipulate this for your own personal body type, and we have seen how to get behind the exact math that comes with knowing how many macros you should be consuming.

We have covered how you can track your macros and some of the easy ways of doing so, we looked at meal planning and the benefits of planning meals in advance (because, let's be honest, it's great being able to eat freely knowing that you already calculated today's macros five days ago), and we have looked at meal combinations that are best for you and your unique body type.

Most importantly, we have learned how to stay motivated, even when falling off the wagon seems like the easy thing to do.

In this book, you have been equipped with a wealth of knowledge that gives you the tools and the power to utilize this weapon for not just weight loss but for a healthier lifestyle too.

Now that you have this power in your hand, go forth and put it into practice. Become the best version of yourself that will ever exist. Let the journey begin!

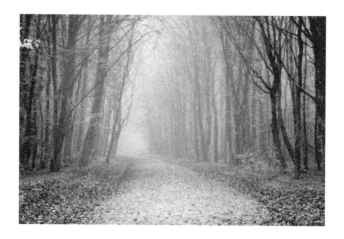

GLOSSARY

- **Carbohydrate:** A macronutrient that serves as a great energy source for humans.
- **Fat:** A macronutrient that is composed predominantly of a greasy or oily matter.
- **Intermittent fasting:** The act of not eating for a period of time, either during the day or over a week. It can be seen as not eating once a week on Tuesdays, or for weight loss purposes, is done on a 16:8 or 18:6 ratio whereby one fasts for 16 hours and eats for a window of six hours in the day.
- **Ketosis:** An innate state of the body whereby fat is used for energy (leading to weight loss) as opposed to glucose which is introduced into the body from food.
- **Macronutrients:** The nutrients that our bodies need in large quantities and that give us the energy we need. Macronutrients fall into three categories, namely carbs, fats, and proteins.
- **Meal preparation:** The act of saving one's future self time and energy by having meals ready to go.
- **Micronutrients:** Nutrients that our bodies need in smaller doses, such as vitamins and minerals.

- **Protein:** A macronutrient that can be found in lean meats or even from some plant sources and that is vital for the repair and building of muscle in the body.
- **Weight loss plateau:** The point in every diet or training plan where the body stops losing weight.

BIBLIOGRAPHY

Abet. (2019, January 24). *Are 800 calorie diets safe?* Scottsdale Weight Loss Center. https://www.scottsdaleweightloss.com/are-800-calorie-diets-safe/

Ajmera, R. (2022, May 27). *Food combinations for weight loss: Do they work?* Healthline. https://www.healthline.com/nutrition/food-combinations-for-weight-loss#weight-loss

Arnold, C. (2010, November 30). *Why diets fail.* Www.science.org. https://www.science.org/content/article/why-diets-fail#:~:text=Changes%20in%20gene%20expression%20may

Avatar Nutrition. (2017, September 9). *At last, the secret to sticking to your diet while traveling or at social events.* https://www.avatarnutrition.com/blog/flexible-dieting/flexible-dieting-traveling-and-social-events

Bhupathiraju, S. N., & Hu, F. (n.d.). *Carbohydrates, protiens, and fats.* Merck Manual. https://www.merckmanuals.com/en-ca/home/disorders-of-nutrition/overview-of-nutrition/carbohydrates,-proteins,-and-fats

Blanton, K. (2022, March 24). *8 scientific benefits of meal prepping.* Everyday Health. https://www.everydayhealth.com/diet-nutrition/scientific-benefits-of-meal-prepping/

Brian Solis quote: *"The distance between who I am and who I want to be is separated only by my actions and words."* (n.d.). Quotefancy.com. https://quotefancy.com/quote/1716240/Brian-Solis-The-distance-between-who-i-am-and-who-i-want-to-be-is-separated-only-by-my

Brueseke, A. (2018, May 30). *5 rookie mistakes beginning macro-trackers make.* Biceps after Babies. https://www.bicepsafterbabies.com/5-rookie-mistakes-beginning-macro-trackers-make/

Calorie Calculator. (n.d.). Www.calculator.net. Retrieved May 28, 2023, from https://www.calculator.net/calorie-calculator.html#:~:text=1%20-pound%2C%20or%20approximately%200.45

Campbell-Danesh, A. (2020, August 31). *Why Do Most Diets Fail in the Long Run?* Psychology Today. https://www.psychologytoday.com/ca/blog/mind-body-food/202008/why-do-most-diets-fail-in-the-long-run

Capritto, A. (2022, December 31). *Instead of calories, you should track this key health metric.* CNET. https://www.cnet.com/health/nutrition/instead-of-calories-you-should-track-this-key-health-metric/

Catudal, P., & Colino, S. (2019, November 18). *Body type quiz: Are you an endomorph, ectomorph, or mesomorph?* EverydayHealth.com. https://www.everydayhealth.com/fitness/do-you-know-your-body-type/

Center for Wellness Without Borders. (n.d.). *The 3 somatotypes*. Www.uh.edu. https://www.uh.edu/fitness/comm_educators/3_somatotypes-NEW.htm#:~:text=William%20H.%20Sheldon%2C%20PhD%2C

Centers for Disease Control and Prevention. (2021, February 11). *Adult obesity facts*. https://www.cdc.gov/obesity/data/adult.html

Clarke, J. (2021, October 7). *Boost confidence and connections by celebrating success the right way*. Verywell Mind. https://www.verywellmind.com/healthy-ways-to-celebrate-success-4163887

Cleveland Clinic. (2022, August 15). *Ketosis: Definition, benefits & side effects*. Cleveland Clinic. https://my.clevelandclinic.org/health/articles/24003-ketosis

Cole, W. (2014, August 5). *7 reasons people fail at weight loss*. Mindbodygreen. https://www.mindbodygreen.com/articles/common-reasons-people-struggle-with-weight-loss#:~:text=Having%20a%20clear%20vision%20of

Collova, A. (2019, September 30). Should I adjust my macros on days that I don't exercise? *IIFYM*. https://www.iifym.com/blog/should-i-adjust-my-macros-on-days-that-i-dont-exercise/

Durand, F. (2019, June 5). *15 tips for better weekly meal planning*. Kitchn. https://www.thekitchn.com/10-tips-for-better-weekly-meal-planning-reader-intelligence-report-177252

Felson, S. (2022, September 27). *14 power pairs for weight loss*. WebMD. https://www.webmd.com/diet/ss/slideshow-food-combos-weight-loss

Field, E. (2022, August 12). *How to adjust your macros: Follow these 3 simple steps*. Emilyfieldrd.com. https://emilyfieldrd.com/blog/simple-steps-to-adjust-your-macros/

Fry, S. (2018, September 7). Ask the dietitian: Are macros important for weight loss? *MyFitnessPal Blog*. https://blog.myfitnesspal.com/ask-the-dietitian-are-macros-important-for-weight-loss/

Gardner, C. D., Trepanowski, J. F., Del Gobbo, L. C., Hauser, M. E., Rigdon, J., Ioannidis, J. P. A., Desai, M., & King, A. C. (2018). Effect of Low-Fat vs Low-Carbohydrate Diet on 12-Month Weight Loss in Overweight Adults and the Association With Genotype Pattern or Insulin Secretion. *JAMA, 319*(7), 667. https://doi.org/10.1001/jama.2018.0245

Gleisberg, L. (2020, June 1). *25 most popular macro tracking questions - answered!* Lauren Gleisberg. https://laurengleisberg.com/popular-macro-tracking-questions-answers/

Gora, A. (2022, July 4). *How to track your macros*. Live Science. https://www.livescience.com/how-to-track-your-macros

Gunnars, K. (2017, May 29). *How protein can help you lose weight naturally*. Healthline. https://www.healthline.com/nutrition/how-protein-can-help-you-lose-weight#TOC_TITLE_HDR_8

Gunnars, K. (2019, March 8). *10 science-backed reasons to eat more protein*. Healthline. https://www.healthline.com/nutrition/10-reasons-to-eat-more-protein#TOC_TITLE_HDR_3

Harvard Health Publishing. (2019). *Eating to boost energy.* Harvard Health. https://www.health.harvard.edu/healthbeat/eating-to-boost-energy

Harvard School of Public Health. (2018, August 15). *Bananas.* The Nutrition Source. https://www.hsph.harvard.edu/nutritionsource/food-features/bananas/#:~:text=One%20serving%2C%20or%20one%20medium

Higuera, V. (2022, January 20). *Endomorph diet: Everything you need to know.* Healthline. https://www.healthline.com/health/food-nutrition/endomorph-diet#diet

Horton, B. (2023, January 18). *We break down everything you need to know about counting macros.* Better Homes & Gardens. https://www.bhg.com/recipes/healthy/eating/what-are-macros/

HSIS. (n.d.). *What happens if people don't get all the vitamins and minerals they need?* HSIS. https://www.hsis.org/did-you-know/what-happens-if-people-dont-get-all-the-vitamins-and-minerals-they-need/#:~:text=There%20are%20now%20strong%20links

Hunt, C. (2021, January 2). *Why counting macros will help you lose weight (and the pitfalls to avoid).* Prospre. https://www.prospre.io/blog/why-counting-macros-will-help-you-lose-weight-and-the-pitfalls-to-avoid

Hyman, M. (2014, May 26). *5 reasons most diets fail (and how to succeed).* Dr. Mark Hyman. https://drhyman.com/blog/2014/05/26/5-reasons-diets-fail-succeed/

Johnson, O. (2020, July 16). *Ectomorph diet: A foolproof way to outwit your genes.* BetterMe Blog. https://betterme.world/articles/ectomorph-diet/

Jomol. (2021, March 2). *12 Common Reasons Why People Fail to Lose Weight.* Makeupandbeauty.com. https://makeupandbeauty.com/common-reasons-why-people-fail-to-lose-weight/#:~:text=Food%20deprivation%20and%20placing%20too

Kallmyer, T. (2021, April 20). *The formula to calculate your macros and REE accurately.* Healthy Eater. https://healthyeater.com/how-to-calculate-your-macros

Katy. (2021, October 4). *When + how should you adjust your macros?* FIT by Katy. https://fitbykaty.com/blogs/fit-blog/when-and-how-to-adjust-macros

Kelly. (2022, December 20). *Learn how to count macros: A beginner's guide.* Eat the Gains. https://eatthegains.com/how-to-count-macros/

Khurshid, H. (2022, June 21). *The history of meal prep - who invented meal preparation?* Marvin's Den. https://marvinsden.com/blogs/all/the-history-of-meal-prep-who-invented-meal-preparation#:~:text=In%20the%201980s%2C%20the%20meal

King, M., & Shiffer, E. (2020, February 26). *"I learned all about macro counting and lost 100 lbs.—and I still ate ice cream every single night."* Women's Health. https://www.womenshealthmag.com/weight-loss/a31045885/counting-macros-drug-addiction-weight-loss-success-story/

Klein, D. (2015, April 1). *Meal frequency and weight loss—is there such a thing as stoking the metabolic fire?* Www.nsca.com. https://www.nsca.com/education/articles/ptq/meal-frequency-and-weight-lossis-there-such-a-thing-as-stoking-the-metabolic-fire/

Knott, A. (2022, December 30). *What macros are right for weight loss?* EatingWell. https://www.eatingwell.com/article/291112/what-macros-are-right-for-weight-loss/

Kollias, H. (2009, February 9). *Body type dieting for ectomorphs, endomorphs, and meso-morphs: Is it right for you?* Precision Nutrition. https://www.precisionnutrition.-com/all-about-body-type-eating#:~:text=Ectomorphs%20were%20thin%2C%20narrow%2C%20delicate

Krans, B. (2015, March 23). *Foods that beat fatigue.* Healthline; Healthline Media. https://www.healthline.com/health/food-nutrition/foods-that-beat-fatigue

Krieger, J. (n.d.). *Counting calories and macros FAQ.* Weightology. https://weightol-ogy.net/online-coaching/counting-calories-and-macros-faq/

LaMeaux, E. C. (n.d.). *How to set a realistic weight loss goal.* Gaiam. https://www.gaiam.-com/blogs/discover/how-to-set-a-realistic-weight-loss-goal

Laskey, J. (2023, January 28). 32 meal planning tips that will make your life easier. Taste of Home. https://www.tasteofhome.com/collection/meal-planning/

Lohman, D. (2016, January 31). *Why can people eat the same diet or take the same medica-tion and have different outcomes?* Morgridge Institute for Research. https://mor-gridge.org/blue-sky/why-can-people-eat-the-same-diet-or-take-the-same-medication-and-have-different-outcomes/#:~:text=Differences%20in%20metabo-lism%20are%20a

Mangano, M. (2016, July 5). *Accountability and weight loss.* Mather Hospital. https://www.matherhospital.org/weight-loss-matters/accountability-and-weight-loss/#:~:text=Weigh%20Yourself%20Regularly%20%E2%80%93%20Knowing%20that

Mayo Clinic. (2018). *Weight loss stalled? Move past the plateau.* https://www.mayoclin-ic.org/healthy-lifestyle/weight-loss/in-depth/weight-loss-plateau/art-20044615

Mayo Clinic. (2021, December 7). *6 proven strategies for weight-loss success.* Mayo Clinic. https://www.mayoclinic.org/healthy-lifestyle/weight-loss/in-depth/weight-loss/art-20047752#:~:text=Set%20realistic%20goals&text=Over%20the%20-long%20term%2C%20it

Mayo Clinic. (2022, October 8). *Can you boost your metabolism?* Mayo Clinic. https://www.mayoclinic.org/healthy-lifestyle/weight-loss/in-depth/me-tabolism/art-20046508#:~:text=Metabolism%20is%20the%20process%20by

Migala, J. (2022a, November 3). *What is the mesomorph diet? Food list, sample menu, benefits, more.* Everyday Health. https://www.everydayhealth.com/diet-nutri-tion/mesomorph-diet/

Migala, J. (2022b, November 6). *What is the ectomorph diet? Food list, sample menu, bene-fits, more.* EverydayHealth.com. https://www.everydayhealth.com/diet-nutri-tion/ectomorph-diet/#:~:text=Ectomorphs%20tend%20to%20respond%20well

Migala, J. (2022c, November 8). *What is the endomorph diet? Food list, sample menu, benefits, more.* Everyday Health. https://www.everydayhealth.com/diet-nutri-tion/endomorph-diet/

Nelson, C. (2021, August 27). *What are macros? Counting proteins, carbohydrates, and fats.* GoodRx. https://www.goodrx.com/well-being/diet-nutrition/how-to-count-macros

Nguyen, D. (2022, March 7). *9 ways to get—and stay—motivated to lose weight.* Forward. https://goforward.com/blog/weight-loss/9-ways-to-get-and-stay-motivated-to-lose-weight#:~:text=But%20it

Olson, R. E. (1998). *Evolution of ideas about the nutritional value of dietary fat: Introduction.* The Journal of Nutrition, 128(2), 421S422S. https://doi.org/10.1093/jn/128.2.421s

Oudeyer, P.-Y., & Kaplan, F. (2007). What is intrinsic motivation? A typology of computational approaches. *Frontiers in Neurorobotics, 1*(6). https://doi.org/10.3389/neuro.12.006.2007

Payne, A. (2020). *Body types: How to train & diet for your body type.* Blog.nasm.org. https://blog.nasm.org/fitness/body-types-how-to-train-diet-for-your-body-type

Pullen, C. (2017, April 24). *16 ways to motivate yourself to lose weight.* Healthline. https://www.healthline.com/nutrition/weight-loss-motivation-tips#TOC_TITLE_HDR_2

Reedy, J. (2021, November 17). *When assessing macros, it's 'quality over quantity' for weight loss.* Blog.insidetracker.com. https://blog.insidetracker.com/assessing-macros-quality-quantity-weight-loss

RUSH. (n.d.). *6 signs of nutrient deficiency.* https://www.rush.edu/news/6-signs-nutrient-deficiency

SA Health. (2020, September 11). *The risks of poor nutrition.* Www.sahealth.sa.gov.au. https://www.sahealth.sa.gov.au/wps/wcm/connect/public+content/sa+health+internet/healthy+living/is+your+health+at+risk/the+risks+of+poor+nutrition#:~:text=In%20the%20short%20term%2C%20poor

Sacks, F. M., Bray, G. A., Carey, V. J., Smith, S. R., Ryan, D. H., Anton, S. D., McManus, K., Champagne, C. M., Bishop, L. M., Laranjo, N., Leboff, M. S., Rood, J. C., de Jonge, L., Greenway, F. L., Loria, C. M., Obarzanek, E., & Williamson, D. A. (2009). Comparison of weight-loss diets with different compositions of fat, protein, and carbohydrates. *The New England Journal of Medicine, 360*(9), 859–873. https://doi.org/10.1056/NEJMoa0804748

Savino, M. (2020, April 8). *Body type & best macros.* Msfitriss.com. https://msfitriss.com/body-type-best-macros/

Sims, S. T. (2016, July 29). *The 3 body types—and how they affect your weight loss.* Prevention. https://www.prevention.com/weight-loss/g20434758/the-3-body-types-and-how-they-affect-your-weight-loss/

Slabaugh, S. (2017, July 4). *How to track macros: A step by step guide for beginners.* Trifecta Nutrition. https://www.trifectanutrition.com/blog/how-to-track-your-macros

Spritzler, F. (2017, February 27). *14 simple ways to break through a weight loss plateau.* Healthline. https://www.healthline.com/nutrition/weight-loss-plateau#TOC_TITLE_HDR_13

10 tips for planning meals on a budget. (2020, November 24). Unlock Food.

https://www.unlockfood.ca/en/Articles/Budget/10-Tips-for-Planning-Meals-on-a-Budget.aspx

United States of America - place explorer. (n.d.). Data Commons. https://datacommons.org/place/country/USA/?utm_medium=explore&mprop=count&popt=Person&hl=en

Van De Walle, G. (2018, September 2). *The best macronutrient ratio for weight loss.* Healthline; Healthline Media. https://www.healthline.com/nutrition/best-macronutrient-ratio#calories-vs-macros

Vetter, C. (2022, January 12). *What to know about macronutrients: Carbs, fat, protein.* Zoe. https://joinzoe.com/learn/carbohydrate-fat-protein-macronutrients

Waehner, P. (2022, June 31). *Setting the right goals for your weight loss success.* Verywell Fit. https://www.verywellfit.com/how-to-set-weight-loss-goals-1231580

Wardleigh, C. (n.d.). *7 benefits of meal prepping.* Select Health. https://selecthealth.org/blog/2019/08/7-benefits-of-meal-prepping

Warshaw, H. (2014, February 4). Q&A: Are meat nutrition labels based on raw or cooked weight? *Washington Post.* https://www.washingtonpost.com/lifestyle/home/qanda-are-meat-nutrition-labels-based-on-raw-or-cooked-weight/2014/02/04/b6f5e2b4-89c0-11e3-916e-e01534b1e132_story.html

WebMD Editorial Contributors. (2021, June 22). *What to know about the mesomorph body type.* WebMD. https://www.webmd.com/fitness-exercise/what-to-know-about-the-mesomorph-body-type#:~:text=Since%20mesomorphs%20tend%20to%20gain

What are macros? A guide to calculating macronutrients for beginners. (n.d.). GrenadeRoW. https://row.grenade.com/blogs/all/a-beginners-guide-to-macros

Williams, C. (2020, June 30). *These are the best times to eat for weight loss, according to a dietitian.* EatingWell. https://www.eatingwell.com/article/7826585/best-times-to-eat-for-weight-loss/

Yu, A. (2022, April 12). *The unspoken weight-discrimination problem at work.* BBC. https://www.bbc.com/worklife/article/20220411-the-unspoken-weight-discrimination-problem-at-work

Zambon, V. (2021, March 8). *Counting macros: What they are, benefits, how to count them.* Medical News Today. https://www.medicalnewstoday.com/articles/how-to-count-macros

Image References

Ahuja, A. (2021). *Woman Measuring her Abdo* [Image]. In Pexels. https://www.pexels.com/photo/woman-measuring-her-abdo-7991934/

Alekseyev, E. (2021). *Roasted meat over a wooden tray* [Image]. In Pexels. https://www.pexels.com/photo/roasted-meat-over-a-wooden-tray-7333166/

Boltneva, V. (2022). *Hamburger with fried meat and chips* [Image]. In Pexels. https://www.pexels.com/photo/hamburger-with-fried-meat-and-chips-11213782/

Brabowska, K. (2020). *Assorted pasta in close-up view* [Image]. In Pexels. https://www.pexels.com/photo/assorted-pasta-in-close-up-view-4039526/

Cowley, N. (2018). *Woman slicing gourd* [Image]. In Pexels. https://www.pexels.com/photo/woman-slicing-gourd-1153369/

Foodie Factor. (2017). *Sliced avocado fruit* [Image]. In Pexels. https://www.pexels.com/photo/sliced-avocado-fruit-557659/

Loring, V. (2020a). *Flatlay of assorted nutritious food* [Image]. In Pexels. https://www.pexels.com/photo/flatlay-of-assorted-nutritious-food-5966434/

Loring, V. (2020b). *Foods in lunch boxes* [Image]. In Pexels. https://www.pexels.com/photo/foods-in-lunch-boxes-5972003/

Maeder, M. (2016). *Red meat with chili pepper and green spies* [Image]. In Pexels. https://www.pexels.com/photo/red-meat-with-chili-pepper-and-green-spies-65175/

Olsson, E. (2018a). *Flat lay photography of three tray of foods* [Image]. In Pexels. https://www.pexels.com/photo/flat-lay-photography-of-three-tray-of-foods-1640775/

Olsson, E. (2018b). *Photo of vegetable salad in bowls* [Image]. In Pexels. https://www.pexels.com/photo/photo-of-vegetable-salad-in-bowls-1640770/

Olsson, E. (2018c). *Three clear glass jars on gray surface* [Image]. In Pexels. https://www.pexels.com/photo/three-clear-glass-jars-on-gray-surface-1640767/

RDNE Stock Project. (2021). *Man in black suit working* [Image]. In Pexels. https://www.pexels.com/photo/man-in-black-suit-working-7821702/

Rebic, I. (2023). *Misty forest road* [Image]. In Pexels. https://www.pexels.com/photo/misty-forest-road-15807415/

RF Studio. (2020). *Crop chemist holding in hands molecule model* [Image]. In Pexels. https://www.pexels.com/photo/crop-chemist-holding-in-hands-molecule-model-3825527/

Riondato, P. (2019). *Pile of red apples* [Image]. In Pexels. https://www.pexels.com/photo/pile-of-red-apples-2966150/

Shvets, A. (2020). *Different body types of woman wearing black clothes* [Image]. In Pexels. https://www.pexels.com/photo/different-body-types-of-woman-wearing-black-clothes-4672237/

Tancredi, L. (2021). *Faceless overweight woman in light clothes* [Image]. In Pexels. https://www.pexels.com/photo/faceless-overweight-woman-in-light-clothes-7065291/

Tankilevitch, P. (2020). *Plate full of fresh vegetables* [Image]. In Pexels. https://www.pexels.com/photo/plate-full-of-fresh-vegetables-4519013/

Thefirst, L. (2020). *Question marks on paper crafts* [Image]. In Pexels. https://www.pexels.com/photo/question-marks-on-paper-crafts-5428829/

Twisty, N. (2020). *Man in white t-shirt and black pants in a running position* [Image]. In

Pexels. https://www.pexels.com/photo/man-in-white-t-shirt-and-black-pants-in-a-running-position-4048182/

Winkler, M. (2020). *Green typewriter on brown wooden table* [Image]. In Pexels. https://www.pexels.com/photo/green-typewriter-on-brown-wooden-table-4052198/

Made in the USA
Columbia, SC
16 September 2023

22963070R00075